LIFE BLOOD

PRAISE FOR

LIFE BLOOD

'This book is a must read for anyone involved in Leukaemia treatment.'
— Geoff Hamilton, AML Survivor

'Cathy's account of her incredible journey is an honour and a privilege to read, reminding us of life's fragility and the importance of 'eyes to the light'. Shared to inspire and help others, her generous and courageous spirit shines all the way through.'
— Susan Mason, The Alfred Foundation.

'Cathy's writing is both personal and refreshingly honest as she explores the good, the bad and the very ugly moments of her cancer journey. If there are questions you always wanted to ask about cancer and treatments but felt awkward doing so, then I suggest you read *Life Blood* — Cathy confronts all topics from hospital food to chemo brain to treatment and recovery with complete frankness and gentle humour.'
— Alex de Fircks, Writer and Blogger

'In spite of all the medical challenges, including a phobia of needles, Cathy's humour shines through in her keen observations of hospital life and the professional staff and volunteers who work tirelessly within the hospital system.

Cathy's thoughtful narration and eloquent language evoke a heartfelt sense of empathy with her struggle to survive and ultimately conquer AML.'
— Jenny Le Boeuf and Tom Landgraf

'*Life Blood* is a bold, honest and heart-warming book, exploring the personal, practical and educational aspects of a journey through a cancer diagnosis and treatment. Cathy's writing is insightful and humorous, emotive and informative; and is a must read. It takes you into her world of the Big C, yet resonates with so many of us who know and love someone impacted by cancer. Full of wise observations and practical tips, *Life Blood* is a fascinating and enlightening insight into the experience of cancer.'

– Danielle Sharkey, Social Worker

'Cathy's story touched my heart. I laughed and cried at this wonderfully written true experience. I could not put it down and would look forward to each chapter, from her factual account of her time with leukaemia to the ironically amusing account of her stay in ICU, where she fantasised about ending it all, and of course so many other wonderful anecdotes. This very real account of Cathy's story is a must read, it is unique yet about something that has affected so many lives.'

– Ronda Baxter

'From the moment she was diagnosed, Cathy refused to give power to the illness – refused to see it as a war in her body that had to be won. *Life Blood* is an intimate expose of Cathy's whole life as much as it is about her experience with the 'little c'. It is written with such insight and humour that it is a joy to read and I laughed out loud many times and was also deeply moved as she shared her extraordinary journey through diagnosis, treatment and the long path to remission and cure.

Life Blood will naturally be of interest to those directly affected by cancer as either a patient or medical professional but also to anyone interested in reading a fellow human's story told with a very bright glint in the authors eye.'

– Tim Browning

'I am very moved by Cathy's telling of her own history. It is such a true and authentic investigation into her journey to survive leukaemia. I have known Cathy for over forty years, and met her shortly after she met her now husband Fred. She has always appeared to me to be a robust, affirmed and sturdy person with a strong sense of self, and it was shattering to her when she was diagnosed with having cancer so unexpectedly and unpreparedly.

Cathy had given herself the challenge to relive and retrace her fight to survive cancer and her ongoing care of herself with repercussions which stay and remain on watch. She presents this investigation as a form of offering of both thanks to all the carers, practitioners, friends and family as much as a way of sharing a very firm belief she has that people need to share individual experiences to build a framework around how they are dealing with their own crises. She offers her story with invitations and challenges, and along with Fred, shares intimate thoughts about life and death. She has come through this journey to share with others who might be struggling with creating a structure around how to survive the many layers of cancer.

It is a multifarious, winding road and Cathy offers important ruminations, questions and reminders. Whether you are a medical student, or someone sitting in a waiting room with a new diagnosis, or someone you know who has a friend who is fighting cancer, this is a very committed and personal journey with lots of ideas and initiatives anyone can use. I commend this special story.'

– Duré Dara OAM

'Cathy's deeply moving story of life threatening cancer and its aftermath is a story of remarkable resilience I take my hat off to anyone who has had to go through anything like this. It is truly wonderful that this book is now out into the world and can make a difference to those who are in the same boat and need some hope.'

– Julie Postance, author of *Breaking the Sound Barriers*

Published in Australia by Silver Moon Press
Postal: PO Box 280 Pyalong Vic 3521
Email: cathykoningwriter@gmail.com
Website: www.cathykoningwriter.com

First published in Australia 2021

National Library of Australia Cataloguing in Publication entry

A catalogue record for this book is available from the National Library of Australia

ISBN 978-0-9943244-1-2 (paperback)
ISBN 978-0-9943244-2-9 (hardcover)
ISBN 978-0-9943244-4-3 (ebook)

Cover design and artwork by Marina Jović
Typesetting by Sophie White Design
Printed by Ingram Spark

Unless otherwise credited, all photographs are from the collection of Cathy Koning

Disclaimer: All care has been taken in the preparation of the information herein, but no responsibility can be accepted by the publisher or author for any damages resulting from the misinterpretation of this work. All contact details given in this book were current at the time of publication, but are subject to change.

The information and opinions expressed in this book are based on the personal experience of the author.The author is not a medical practitioner and the recommendations given in this book are solely intended as education and information of a general nature. The book is not designed to provide diagnosis or treatment or any type of professional medical advice. If you or any other individual choses to take any recommendations from this book, please do not do so before consulting your health care professional.

LIFE BLOOD

Lessons from one woman who survived
serious illness against the odds

CATHY KONING

This book is dedicated to all the amazing, compassionate and professional staff at Melbourne's Alfred Hospital, recognised as one of the world's leading hospitals.

CONTENTS

Foreword   13

Introduction   15

One   Who am I?   21

Two   Something's wrong   43

Three   Let the Treatment Begin   49

Four   ICU – I see you, but not very well   83

Five   Life after ICU – Rehabilitation   103

Six   The stem cell transplant   109

Seven   What else can go wrong?   115

Eight   Why Me?   139

Nine   It's all in the mind   147

Ten   Becoming a Carer – Fred's thoughts   163

Eleven   Things that pulled me through   171

Twelve   Who am I now?   189

Some Practical Advice for Patients and Carers   213

Useful contacts   225

Further reading   227

Acknowledgments   229

About the author   231

FOREWORD

As a doctor, one of the hardest things you have to do is tell someone they have cancer. The effect of the word is instant and profound: it strikes terror deep into the heart. If you – or someone you love – have been given this diagnosis, you know exactly what I mean. The shock is profound. It's an assault to the senses. It's almost impossible to take in; to get your head around this frightening new reality, and the dreadful uncertainty that goes with it. Your mind spins in circles: What does this mean? What do you need to do? Where do you turn to? What happens next? I trust this book will be of great comfort to anyone facing such difficulties.

I've known Cathy Koning for many years; her husband, Fred, was the first friend I made when I emigrated to Australia 30 years ago. In these pages, she has written an honest, moving, and real account of her 'close encounter' with leukaemia – which I remember all too vividly. It was such a shock to me, to see Cathy lose all her hair, waste away to almost nothing, struggle to even move in her bed... and such a great delight when she eventually pulled through.

And although Cathy's story is about leukaemia, her experiences are deeply relatable for any type of cancer: her fears, her struggles, her desperation, her obstacles, her courage, and her commitment. This book will give you a good idea of what you (or a loved one) may go through when facing cancer. It's a heart-warming account of a heroic journey. And it offers a message of courage and hope for all. I trust you will find it both a source of valuable information and a comfort amidst times of great suffering.

— Dr Russ Harris, Melbourne, 2021

INTRODUCTION

Five years after my leukaemia diagnosis Professor Curtis asks how I am feeling. I reply, 'I have never been so unhappy.' I tell him about my illness de jour. I see his face fall.

Not for the first time I contemplate how he copes with patients like me when we are feeling scared and sorry for ourselves. Medical staff aim to give us their best care and advice, nevertheless this cancer racket can make a person so self-obsessed and oh-so self-indulgent. Doctors (and nurses) are trained to deal with the science first. They are in the healthcare business and choose to be surrounded by us sooky sickies. If I was a doctor I would become sick and tired of downcast patients who keep on asking what their chances of survival are and probably expect the worst, and let's face it, leukaemia doesn't offer the best survival rates for older people. Still, it must be hard to break bad news... No, the treatment isn't working. Yes, you have reached the end of the line kiddo. Your karma is not great. Maybe you will have better luck in your next life... The satisfaction must be in seeing us cancer survivors, us valiant warriors, sticking around, even if it is to pester the hell out of our doctors and nurses by occasionally feeling sorry for ourselves.

Medical professionals do receive training in breaking bad news, in grief counselling and how to cope with emotionally charged situations. And they do need to find their own particular way of dealing compassionately with those of us who are facing a bleak prognosis.

When Dr Michael Dickinson, a clinical haematologist, was interviewed about this topic by Hannie Rayson for *The Age* he said, 'It's not something I shy away from, but there have been a few situations this year where I've had to stand up and leave because I was about to burst into tears. I didn't want to do that. In front of people. Particularly young people, with their parents in the room. My way of coping is this: Yes, the patient is scared. They want to talk and be heard. But mostly they want to survive. They want an expert. They want you to get it right. The right treatment. The best advice. I hope I don't sound like a robot telling you this,' he says, 'but my coping mechanism is just to be good at what I do.'*

Welcome to the roller coaster world of Acute Myeloid Leukaemia (AML)

I want to share my experience for all of you who want to know more about cancer from a patient's point of view. I hope it will inform others who are facing a similar path and want to know what may lie ahead, help caregivers support their friend or family member and encourage medical professionals to look beyond the disease to the person. I believe understanding the patient will help inform the management of their disease. The type of treatment and level of support required is very individualised so it makes sense to take time to investigate the person. This is particularly the case with cancer as the relationship between patient and doctor is often maintained over many years. My Professor has been managing my case for nine years and counting.

Acute Myeloid Leukaemia seems to be a particularly insidious cancer as a stem cell transplant may remove the cancer from your body but managing the effects of the transplant can bring many unforeseen and unpredictable side effects. Being cured can feel like a victory but it does not mean back to business as usual. For me recovery has not been a single line from diagnosis to medical intervention to feeling better and thanks, see you later. The cancer train stops at many stations. It has been a series of setbacks and recoveries which have gone on much longer than you would expect after being cured. These

---

* Hannie Rayson 'Life at the Cancer Coalface: My coping device is just to be good at what I do.' *The Age*, 26 January, 2019, p. 20

have included the initial chemotherapy; developing sepsis resulting in over three weeks in an Intensive Care Unit (ICU); the actual stem cell transplant; graft vs host disease (GVHD) which can often occur after the transplant; shingles; type 2 diabetes; pneumonia and the challenging side effects of the drugs you need to take to manage the side effects of treatment.

Cancer is a remarkable teacher, a life-changing learning experience. To a large extent it is all about the numbers. It does take work to achieve the good readings. Years of work in my case. I have been asked if the journey, or expedition as I like to call it, has been worthwhile. Definitely. I am grateful to still be 100% alive. But I haven't always felt this way. Although rewarding in ways I never expected, being a cancer patient can be challenging, taxing and energy sapping too. Sometimes a change of terminology can help. I decide to call my cancer the little c rather than the Big C. I'm not giving it that much power!

Today

There are no guarantees, but for now I am feeling well.

I'm sitting at my writing desk, looking out the window and making a note of what I see. It is all happening in my haven. The view expands out to farmland, all dry, brown and yet gorgeous in the Australian summer heat. A row of blindingly white tee-shirts hang from the makeshift clothesline strung up between two blue gums. A mob of kangaroos stops by, alternatively grazing and staring intently. One has a little joey poking its head out of the pouch and two of the young roos are having a little boxing match. Galahs, whose pink, cream and grey feathers remind me of the colours in a 1950s formica table, drink at the bird bath. Baby magpies squawk nonstop while their parents show them how to find worms. White cockatoos hang upside down off a seeding wattle bush like fat Christmas ornaments. A thrush sings a delicious melody, up and down the scales, perfectly in tune. Meanwhile our tabby cat, Gus, naps in the sun, enjoys a dust bath and then demands a back scratch from my husband Fred.

I revisit this book's chapter describing the sojourn in ICU. I tell Fred I started crying after rereading the emails he sent during that awful time.

Accepting the changes

I cry easily these days. A while ago I attended a performance of Mahler's *Ninth Symphony* in San Francisco and surprised myself by quietly weeping right through the final movement. It is difficult to put the feelings Mahler's music evokes into words. Whatever regrets or grief Mahler may have had at this time in his life, only a few years from his own death, seem to disappear, giving way to peace and silence. I thought of my mother taking her last breath. I couldn't help but feel quite melancholy. My dear friend Paulette, who we were staying with, happened to be a nurse who worked with blood cancer patients. She offered some wise words to me. 'The past is past. It is like a cancelled cheque and the future is yet to come. If you are dreading and dreaming about the future, you are missing what is here now.'

The future

Will I be around to see further positive change? I certainly hope so. The chances of the AML returning are statistically small thanks to my donor stem cell transplant. That's the good news. I don't worry too much about getting sick again. I'll deal with it at the time. If the worst happens, I will hop right back to Melbourne's Alfred Hospital and see what they can do for me. As to the future, like most of us I hope to live out my days at home, eating well and enjoying life surrounded by lush native foliage and watching cockatoos from my back veranda. This could be unrealistic but fingers crossed.

Cancer *does* change your life, without a doubt. For better, for worse. For richer, for poorer. And I cannot deny, and don't want to deny, the many wonderful (and challenging) experiences I have had since AML came into my life and I want to recount some of them for you. For patients who are confronted with a life-threatening illness I want to share my story to show you there will be bad days but there are also good ones and some of my experiences may help you through. Although I do challenge certain perceptions, I don't have a particular barrow to push. Your thoughts and insights about cancer may be quite different to mine, and just as valid. Everyone has to meet the challenge of illness in their own way.

There are many things family and friends can do to help. I have included what worked for me. I offer show and tell, ideas for you to compare and contrast, along with some practical advice. For medical professionals I hope to give you a glimpse into the world of one patient and the strengths and fears I brought to my treatment.

ONE

———

Who am I?

Medical practitioners, when confronted with a seriously ill patient, generally turn to their science-based training to diagnose and treat the patient's disease. However, taking some time to get to know their patient can also assist with the management of their treatment. Every person sitting in a doctor's waiting room or occupying a hospital bed has life experiences, personality traits and a family history which will determine how they respond to a serious illness such as cancer.

So who am I and what did I bring with me in my encounter with cancer?

Family

My parents, Anne and Theodorus (Dick), were Dutch immigrants who came to Australia in the 1950s. My dad was a horticulturist who had worked in glasshouses so the government found him work on a sheep station in central New South Wales where I was born. I have two younger brothers, Peter and John. Mum and Dad were hard working and, as a result, our

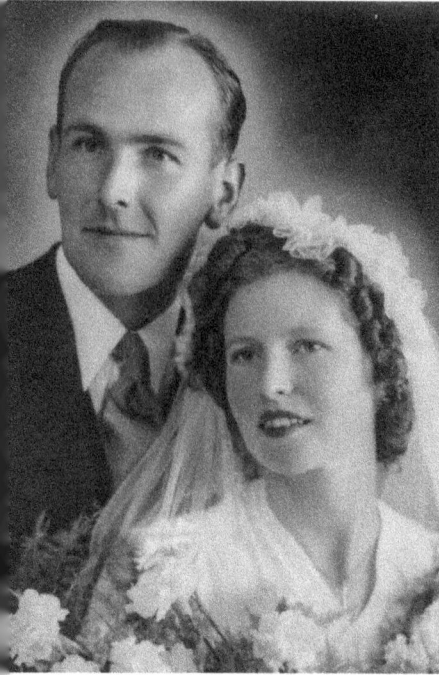

Above; Anne and Dick on their Wedding day. Below; Leaving Amsterdam for Sydney by KLM Lockheed Constellation.

family moved house many times in search of better job opportunities. With the enlargement of the Eildon Weir in 1961, a Rural Finance Closer Settlement irrigation area was opened in northern Victoria comprising one hundred and seventy irrigated dairy and orchard holdings. My parents were fortunate enough to be allocated an orchard of peaches, pears and apricots numbered block 42. This is where I lived from the age of ten until I left for Melbourne's La Trobe University where, at eighteen, I took up a teaching studentship and met Fred.

In the early 1970s there was a shortage of secondary teachers in regional areas. The Victorian Government funded my Bachelor of Arts degree in History/Sociology and

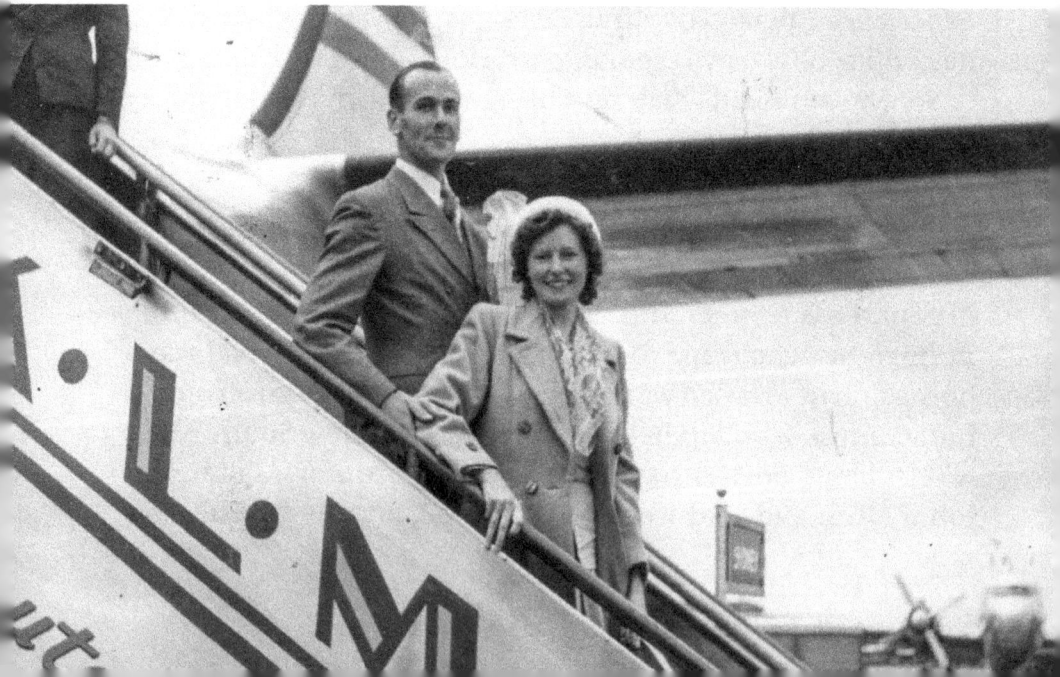

a Diploma of Education in exchange for a commitment to teach for three years. After my three years were up I decided to resign from teaching. At this time Fred commenced a career in theatre production which gave me the opportunity to photograph shows. I also toured Europe as photographer with *Momma's Little Horror Show*, a brilliant mix of puppetry, magic and black theatre created by Nigel Triffitt.

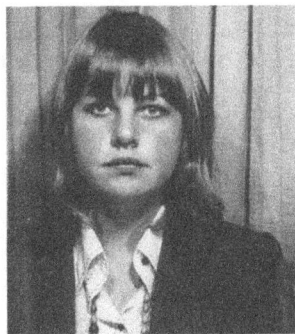

1969 – looking cool at 17 years of age.

Over the years my resume reflected my deep interest in cinema, with stints working front of house at Hoyts and as a publicist for a leading arthouse cinema. However, working indoors with no windows to gaze out of began to pall. I told one of the film reviewers I planned to become a gardener; one of those crazy light bulb moments. He said, 'My garden needs work.' So off I went, using my pseudo-sporty orange Datsun 180B as a mouldy work vehicle, and reinvented myself as a horticulturist. I met Fran and together we founded Your Gardening Angels, concentrating on the sustainable maintenance of gardens in some of Melbourne's affluent suburbs. Fred and I then moved to the country, just outside Melbourne, where we purchased a house in 2004.

After a stint of casual relief teaching I was employed by two local shires to run their Sustainable Communities Program. The three-year workshop-based program offered a splendid opportunity for me as it brought together my skills as an educator, publicist, photographer and horticulturalist. Around this time Fred worked at Monash University which was too far to commute from our home. So, in exchange for working some nights and weekends as a boarding master at Xavier College, a private boys school, he lived in a small flat in the boarding house. There was a great deal of travelling between the country and city. By December 2011 my community program was successfully completed so Gus the cat and I moved in with him. Xavier would become my unlikely, but safe, haven.

On 29 March 2012, a date etched into my memory, I was diagnosed with Acute Myeloid Leukaemia.

Am I Dying?

Death seems to be the first thing you think about with this diagnosis.

Immediately after my diagnosis I found myself in The Alfred's Emergency Department. I floundered around on the narrow hospital bed and dredged up dozens of euphemisms about death from the depths of my mind to distract myself from sounds and smells of the other emergency patients parked in their curtained cubicles. I like descriptions with a gangster edge; you can never watch enough film noir – rubbed out, bumped off, swimming with concrete shoes, feeding the fishes and wearing a pine overcoat.

For the theatricals, of whom there are many in my circle, we have: curtains, fading to black, taking a last bow and climbing the golden staircase. Botanically inclined? Pushing up daisies has a nice floral ring to it. What about six feet under? Carpenters may prefer dead as a doornail, wearing wooden pyjamas or another nail in the coffin. Duke Ellington's *Take the A Train* for the jazz and railway aficionados?

I could go on, and on. Why not? I'm not so sure about passing away as a description of death, although it does remind me of ships passing each other and slowly getting smaller as they disappeared from view.

I do like disappeared. Maybe that is what will happen to me. Disappearing into the sunset, never to be seen again.

There were no, why me? moments at this stage. My question was, Why not me?

An experience of death – losing my mother

We all bring our own experience of death to fearful situations.

Seven months after I experienced my first symptoms my mother chose her time to die, or so I like to think. She knew her time had come to let go. A few years before, we were chatting on the phone about getting older and the inevitability of death, as you do. She told me to live my life to the full and not to mourn too much or for too long when she passed.

Mum was pragmatic to the last. At the nursing home the elderly people were lined up against the wall, asleep in their chairs. Dead to the world. I will never forget Mum's words 'Look at those people just sitting there unconscious. There is no way I'm going to end up like them. No way.' And she was as good as her word. So she chose to shut down her bodily functions. She stopped eating and hardly drank any liquids.

As Mum aged, I made a resolution that we would not have any unresolved issues between us before she died but there are still regrets. I have too many regrets to mention, and I bet I am not alone. Is there such a thing as closure after a loved one dies? I don't believe so, for myself anyway.

After Mum died she was cremated. Some of her ashes were placed in the family grave near Shepparton and Fred and I later took the remainder with us to The Netherlands. The eldest of ten children, Mum grew up in a small village surrounded by canals. Three of her siblings settled in Australia and two sisters and one brother were still living in The Netherlands. The catholic church where my parents were married is surprisingly large; solid as a rock, made of finely detailed brick and quite beautiful. We added Mum's ashes to the family grave, returning a small part of her back to her home town; a poignant moment.

Time to think about religion. As you do after you nearly die.

Belief

One day in a taxi, returning from post-ICU rehabilitation I noticed the driver had a religious program playing on the radio. He asked me if I believed in God. You should have seen his face when I replied 'no' to annoy him. I ended up paying the driver for his intrusive preaching in addition to the privilege of being taken from A to B. I did not have the energy to convey my experiences or my real thoughts about cancer, God and spirituality with him.

Before I became ill my ideas regarding death and religion were somewhat underdeveloped. I did not talk often in any depth about death with my family or friends. Every now and then, especially after my father died, I contemplated if there was life after death. I couldn't come up with any satisfactory answers and tried to put it out of my mind.

I was brought up a catholic. Mum and Dad were both lapsed catholics before they died. As a child I loved to go to our tiny country church on a Sunday, checking out our priest in full vestments of lace and satin; the embroidered silks with the IHS logo on them; the intense, heady perfume of the incense; the romantic words spoken in Latin. But much of what I was taught about God made no sense, in Latin, English or otherwise. The concept of God creating the earth in seven days did my head in. I learned Adam was given dominion over the animals and the earth. (Big mistake; the genesis of exploitation and environmental disaster right there.) I do not subscribe to the concept of punishment and reward in the next life as the priests and nuns taught it. Or the idea of purgatory as some sort of soul parking spot before we can reach heaven (or hell). But I do think Jesus was a special, powerful person.

The cancer experience has not affected the way I think about dying. I have not had my beliefs clarified or undergone a spiritual epiphany. When I came out of the induced coma in ICU I believed there was no life after death. I do not find solace in the christian concept of religion. It is so male dominated. Even God is male – father, son and Holy Ghost. That does not give meaning to my life. But I do believe in energy being transformed, before and after death. Being in the garden or at the beach gives me that sense of energy. I like the thought of our energy or life force transforming after we die. We are tiny little specs of star stuff after all. I subscribe to the theory of evolution over the millennia, the big bang, the expanding universe. At thirteen I had an overwhelming experience. One hot summer's night *Dr Who* was on the TV battling with a selection of giant maggot-like creatures. They made a high-pitched buzzing sound which matched the noise the crickets were making outside. I sat on our front veranda and looked up at the myriad stars cluttering up the sky, contemplating the concept of infinity. And quietly had a small brain meltdown. I could not understand it. How could anything not have an end? I felt anxious and sick for days. However, I did not ask my parents or teachers for help. I now think everything has a beginning and an end, even the universe.

I did ask Mum why sex before marriage and killing someone were both mortal sins, sins which could send you to hell. Those sins are not all that original and certainly not equal in my eyes. And, if God did exist, if God is all-loving, what was the point of all the suffering in the world? Did God send us cancer as a punishment? What is the point of the pain cancer causes?

Belief in God, and in prayer, can certainly be comforting. While I was in hospital a priest said a prayer over me. At a friend's request, the Buddhist monks in Bendigo included me on their prayer list and prayers were said at Xavier during Sunday mass. I was grateful to receive them. But why, given my beliefs? Having prayers said for you is a loving action. Others are sending out positive energy, focussing on you. It is calming.

Every person who experiences cancer will have their own personal response – managing their deepest fears of losing everything, the unknown, facing death. I have seen comments by survivors wondering how anyone can get through cancer without having God in their lives. After completing the first draft of this book I came across a blog by local man, Geoff Hamilton, entitled *Geoff Beats Leukemia* which he started after being diagnosed with Acute Myelomonocytic Leukaemia, a subgroup of AML, in August 2017. His thoughts on cancer, resilience and spirituality struck a chord with me:

I would say that I like to live my life according to the principles of mankind – kindness, helpfulness, acceptance etc. etc. These are key principles and they are not owned by any one religion. I do believe I am a person of spirituality as there are many things of beauty, love and relationships that science cannot explain. (But a specific religion does not have a monopoly…)

So if I were to follow the science line then I am much more comfortable with my condition and how people get sick.

In this game the doctors measure absolutely everything. Fluids in, fluids out, drugs in, blood tests regularly (up to 3 times a day) and blood culture tests for virus development. Nurses check blood pressure, body temperature and heart rate, blood oxygen levels every few hours (makes it hard to get sleep of course).

Treating cancer is a process. Once all the measurements are in and the Medical Team (it is certainly not just one doctor making all the decisions) review the data they start pulling levers and managing the outcomes. They know what to expect in general terms having delivered similar treatments many times before and of course relying on the extensive worldwide scientific papers and reviews of similar treatments. They are highly intelligent people who are well trained and well meaning. For me they are my God.

So while I may not believe in the artificial construct of a formal religion, I do have my own personal set of beliefs that suit me and provide me with comfort.

What about a funeral party?

Thinking about death leads to the inevitable thoughts about my funeral. I have attended quite a few funerals, ranging from the mundane to the inspired, and started thinking about how I wanted my own event staged. Lately I have been day-dreaming, conjuring up ideas for favourite songs to be played. Any thoughts for some retro tunes?

How about Led Zeppelin's, *In My Time of Dying*, a phenomenal rendition of an old blues song from the deep south of America? Might be a test for the attendees at eleven minutes though. I came up with an even better idea; instead of a funeral let's have a party before I push up daisies, as long as I'm not too sick to enjoy it. It could provide an opportunity for everyone to catch up. Family and friends with a few nice words to say or a stock of amusing anecdotes to share are most welcome to join in. Perhaps Fred can organise the food, the flowers and the music. He has a background in event management after all. I'm thinking curries, pink carnations (I love the spicy cinnamon-like perfume they emit), mimosa cocktails, local craft beer and Led Zeppelin interspersed with a short, carefully considered selection from Gustav Mahler's ten glorious symphonies and *Beim Schlafengehen (When Falling Asleep)*, the third of the *Four Last Songs* by Richard Strauss.

Like Mum and Fred's mother, Thelma, I plan to be cremated. Wrap me in calico like my cats, Tabby and Furry, after they died and select a simple, inexpensive cardboard coffin for the guests to write on. I would like some of my ashes to be spread under a yellow box gum tree in the garden.

I hate hospitals

Quite an important thing to know about me – as a result of a number of events in my life, especially as a child – I hate medical procedures and hospitals.

I had managed to steer away from having a blood test since 1976 but I did require the occasional vaccination and procedure as an adult. Why the avoidance? Because undergoing any kind of injection, putting any substance into my arm or taking any substance out, was terrifying, leading to sweating, panic attacks and insomnia. At times I came close to passing out just visiting a patient in hospital, and once, on admittance to hospital for a short stay, the receptionist asked for my address but I could not remember where I lived. The memory department of my brain had frozen. My mother said she never worried about me trying heroin; beauty procedures such as botox were never top of my bucket list. For our ancestors crouching in their caves, having punctured skin and running the risk of infection was a real threat to life. That fear made total sense to me.

There are different types of fear of needles or trypanophobia; some sufferers fear the sight, thought or feel of needles, have experienced or witnessed a traumatic medical event, or have had prior procedures with forced physical or emotional restraint. I'm proud to say, or should I say sad to say, I fit every category on the needle phobia list. This made me an excellent candidate for a lifetime of avoidance of healthcare and medical procedures. This fact would of course have a huge impact psychologically during my treatment.

It started with tonsils

Even though they are a significant part of the immune system, doctors were mad for taking out tonsils at the first sign of recurrent infection in the 1950s. It was fashionable but often unwarranted. I was not quite four-years-old when I underwent the operation at the local hospital. This was probably fortunate; I have read of children being operated on at home on the kitchen table. Remarkably, I can still remember what happened. Mum and Dad were kind and told me what to expect, in very broad terms. Ice cream was mentioned as a treat after the deed had been done.

I was calm until the hospital staff placed me on the operating table when all hell then broke loose. The doctors and nurses were attempting to murder me (or so I thought). They were trying to hold me down for a start. It was a fight to the death. I fought and punched and tried to escape. 'Here's a little blanket for you little girl,' the doctor said. I kicked the blanket off with all my might and maybe kicked him in the crotch too. Hands came from everywhere to force me down; the ether was placed on a cloth inside a mask and pushed onto my face and that is all

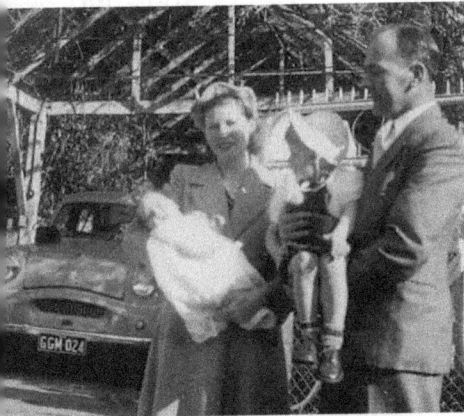

My family with the new Standard 8. Dandenong Victoria.

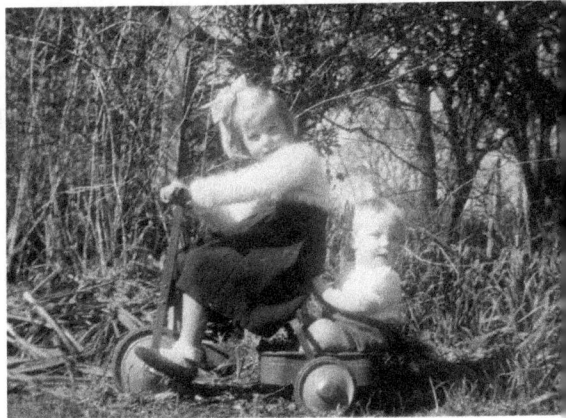

With Peter not long before my tonsil operation.

I remembered. Afterwards, although the ice cream was tasty, I had great difficulty swallowing because my throat was so sore. I felt drained, defeated and exhausted. Something changed inside me. I did not want to see the inside of a hospital ever again and that feeling never went away. My body retained an implicit memory of what I perceived as an assault. A few years ago I saw a display of old medical implements at my local hospital including the metal gadget used for cutting the tonsils. Seeing it nearly made me faint.

Almost losing my mother

Around the time of my tonsillectomy another operation saved my mother from excruciating pain and saved her life. A blockage had developed in a tube leading to her kidneys. A frightening situation. I remember Mum writhing on the bed in absolute agony but there was nothing I could do to make her pain go away. At Melbourne's St Vincent's Hospital the surgeons inserted a small plastic tube and like magic – her kidney flow was all fixed. The technology was new; a few years earlier there would have been little they could do. My mother would have died, Dad would have been bereft and my brother and I left without our mother's love and care. So two traumatic medical procedures at a similar time during my formative years had a profound effect on my psyche and lay the foundation for greater trepidation in the years to come.

Then there was measles

A short time later, I must have been around six, I developed pneumonia as a complication from measles. There were no vaccinations for measles in those days. Another medical horror show was in store for me, although also a lifesaving experience thanks to penicillin. The needles used for delivering said lifesaver into my buttocks were huge, metallic and painful. I commenced to weep in terror every time the nurse came along with the metal kidney dish, before she had even done the deed. It must have been awful for her too. Don't cry little girl, said the boy in the bed next to me, but I couldn't help it.

Are you starting to get the picture...?

It's immunisation time

Regular needles at school for diseases such as tuberculosis completed the phobia job. These injections were given without finesse. A case of line up, pull up your sleeve and quietly face the jab – next arm please. The same needle was used for the entire class; we all lined up in alphabetical order. Having the surname of Koning, the needle was only half blunt by the time my turn arrived. One or two kids cried or fainted; others didn't feel a thing and some did not turn up at all. A thump on the arm from a classmate helped round off the experience.

Teeth extractions

Another scary experience happened in the mid-1960s, this time at the dentist. In my teenage years my teeth grew too big for my mouth (something to do with evolution and eating less meat). We could not afford the cost of braces so the removal of a few pearly white teeth was the only option. The dentist's darkly lit surgery was so primitive that a diploma from the 1920s still featured on his wall. All his tools of trade, including the dentist chair upholstered in faux brown leather, seemed to be from that era too, akin to entering a medical museum.

The combined effect of my tonsillectomy, helplessly watching my mother in pain, injections, immunisations and teeth extractions created a whole lot of angst and resulted in the avoidance of anything medical.

A victim of white coat syndrome?

Sometimes, while visiting a medical clinic, my anxiety has resulted in blood pressure readings being much higher than normal. This is termed white coat syndrome.

My fear of injections was not a secret in my family, just a fact of life. Cathy's scared of needles. No-one ever suggested I should seek out help, or even get over it. Seeing a therapist was not on the radar and sitting around delving deeply into emotional issues did not happen. My family could not afford the cost of therapy anyway. I was born with a silver-plated spoon in my mouth, not a hallmarked solid silver one. Nevertheless, understanding my deep-rooted fear of medical procedures would have helped the medical professionals who I saw in my younger days do their job more effectively.

My community

On the positive side, my cancer experience certainly did not happen in a vacuum.

I received beautiful messages of support full of encouragement and love. My friends and family are so wise; a large network of kind and thoughtful people and an amazing partner supported me each step of the way. The encouraging emails, texts, gifts, messages on Fred's Facebook page and cards made me feel that the people in my circle were much better friends to me then I had been to them over the years.

My cousin Maria, whom I have known all my life, wrote about how much she valued our relationship.

'It's impossible to imagine what you are feeling and going through but you have resilience and have been through dark times before. You can do this. Each time I write down something it doesn't seem quite right in the circumstances. On the one hand daily goings on are so trite given what you

are dealing with. On the other, the things I want to say as words of encouragement and love sound like goodbyes but that's not what they are. Cathy, I have never said how much I value your presence in my life and how deeply grateful I am for our family relationship, our friendship and our shared journey. I just want you to know that.'

The message from my mother was especially moving because she said how much she loved me.

'It is indeed a horrible thing to have to go through. It really is incredible. It shows you never know what's in store for anybody. Do you remember your Dad saying, 'It doesn't matter what your plans are, somebody or something is sure to bugger it up.' Ain't that the truth!

Well darling, all I can say is try to keep a positive outlook on things... Your greatest positive is called Fred, if there is such a thing as lucky in a case like yours, I can't emphasise enough how lucky you are to have him.'

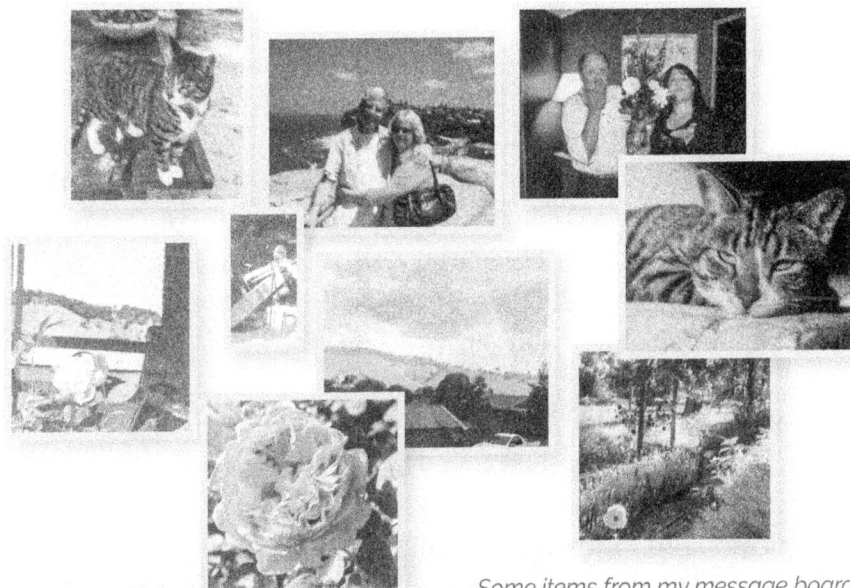

Some items from my message board.

Too true. Tears flowed.

The little flat at Xavier College turned out to be a totally supportive place. I reclined on the couch all day knowing the boarding staff, cafeteria staff and boarders were about. They were there as needed but did not intrude. A private boys' school was an unusual environment in which to recover from cancer. I could hear the Xavier students going about their day, chatting away. It was very comforting. The year twelve boarders brought me a lovely bunch of pink lilies. To say I appreciated this gesture is an understatement. One of the boarders who grew up in the remote Western Australian town of Broome shared an essay about his deep love for the beach; the calm feeling when he put his head underwater and watched the air bubbles rise, the sand between his toes and the sun on his back. His beautiful words had a healing effect.

Having a community to support both Fred and me had a huge influence on my ability to cope with the treatment.

Fred

We were always planning a big party when I turned sixty, but we celebrated by getting married instead. A big afternoon tea was planned in June with family and friends but when the time came I was still in hospital and not up to celebrating. By then Fred and I had lived together for thirty-seven years. If anyone asked why we had not yet married, one of us would reply, 'Actually I'm not sure. I don't think I'm ready.' Mum called Fred her sin-in-law.

We first met at La Trobe University in 1975. I was in the final year of my BA, Dip Ed and Fred was running the STA travel office at the university. He had studied social work at Melbourne University but changed careers after seeing one too many clients in Pentridge Prison.

I liked Fred immediately. He had thick, curly brown hair,

although it was a bit unkempt in those days. He was easy to talk to and has a good sense of humour. He usually wore a black velvet jacket with flared denim jeans patched in various fabrics. I ran around in vintage crepe and lace evening dresses from the 1930s paired with black lace up boots during the day. I thought I was cool.

Fred has spent most of his working life in the arts on the production side. His idea of happiness is attending a performance of one of Gustav Mahler's symphonies anywhere in the world and I have been delighted to go with him. We have heard Mahler played by top orchestras in New York, Amsterdam, Leipzig, London and around Australia. Travel and stimulating experiences in general have been high on our agenda.

By the time we married only one parent was still there to celebrate with us. Both our fathers had died in 1981. Dad died suddenly of heart disease at the age of sixty-two; Fred's father Reg died as a result of health problems initially triggered by

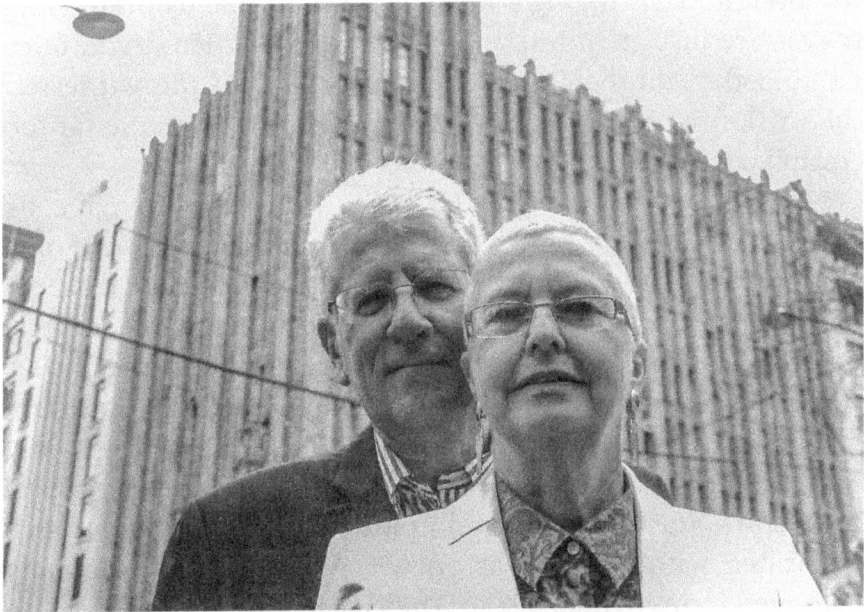

Taken on our wedding day. Photograph by Rod Scanlan.

service in New Guinea during the Second World War. Mum and Fred's mum, Thelma, became firm friends and health discussions were regularly a focus of their chats. I told Fred I did not want to talk to my friends about my poor physical condition when I reached old age and he agreed. Famous last words. Thelma died in 2004 at the age of eighty-seven.

As my sixtieth birthday approached, according to the latest bone marrow biopsy I was still technically in remission after two rounds of chemo. That did not mean I was feeling fit. Far from it. My energy level was low, not the normal tiredness which dissipates after a good night's sleep. More like a permanent veil over my vitality, a veil you hope will lift but sticks around and becomes part of your daily life.

Fred and I decided to get married. We had not needed to tie the knot before but now it felt right. So on 26 August 2012 we turned my birthday party into a wedding; a small ceremony at the Westin Hotel in the city in front of sixty guests before we all enjoyed a delicious afternoon tea. At first we thought of springing a surprise on everyone by pretending they were just attending my birthday party. However, once we told the immediate family and organised the witnesses, the work involved in keeping the event secret became far too complicated and ultimately unnecessary.

No, I didn't wear a big meringue-style dress or have six bridesmaids. I spent hours shopping for an outfit but the only clothes I liked were a Paul Smith shirt at $600 and a jacket at $1300. As my friend Fran said, 'Rolls Royce taste on a bicycle income,' my income had shrunk to zero due to the little c putting me out of employment. Fred and I did scrub up alright for the occasion. He wore a suit and I was pleased with my Marcs light pink jacket paired with a William Morris inspired print shirt. For something old I pinned a delicate gold brooch decorated with seed pearls onto the lapel. It had originally belonged to my Oma back in The Netherlands.

I noticed Mum seemed a bit tired and a little out of it during the event. In addition to the minor stroke she had experienced, the bones in one of her hips had deteriorated over the years which meant she couldn't walk far without pain.

Our friend Jim cancelled all his business appointments and jumped on a plane from San Francisco to attend the wedding. He said he couldn't stay away. My cousin Maria flew in from Brisbane and Frank from Perth.

There was a great outpouring of emotion during the ceremony. All the guests were either family or close friends of many years standing. We shared a history. We knew each other's foibles, shared life's ups and downs, had gone on trips and worked together, leading to many humorous moments too.

I did not have the energy to think fully about the details. Duré and David came to the rescue with the gift of a bridal bouquet of tulips and an exquisite two-tiered wedding cake, created by leading Sydney cake artist and friend Anthea who also came to the event. Fred and I both gave a small speech. This wedding was not like most others. We had been together for thirty-seven years, did not have any offspring, had lived in eleven houses, had lost count of the number of jobs we had worked and attended around 200 family events. The AML added a poignant air – it was essential to acknowledge publicly what my family went through, the trust they had put in Fred and to thank all our buddies for their support. I was totally over the focus on me and my health but gave an update anyway. I told everyone I fancied myself as the great survivor. Things could go either way as I was not yet cured.

Fred spoke about how his love grew over time; he wrote in an email to everyone that he had fallen in love with me all over again when I was in hospital. I talked about our relationship being strong enough to meet the obstacles we had faced over the years.

I chose a poem from Rumi, the 13th century Persian poet and mystic, and Fred read the Clara Schumann poem, *If you Love for Beauty*.

A holiday followed at Mission Beach in Queensland where we rented a house right on the beach. The devastation from Cyclone Yasi was still very much in evidence. We saw two cassowaries (but no crocodiles or jelly fish), ate hotdogs, drank coffee on the beach and bought local seafood from the market. We also played Scrabble every day and sat around looking out to sea. I started to feel more positive about the future.

Be positive

Is too much emphasis on positive thinking placed on the cancer patient? Does an optimistic attitude help when the little c comes knocking? Can positive thinking cure cancer? Hmmm. Was Monty Python's Eric Idle correct to *Always Look on the Bright Side of Life* in the worst of circumstances? What about the power of pragmatic thinking?

While my father was at heart a kindly man, he was introverted and did not find it easy to share his feelings; Mum was outwardly more upbeat, more hopeful. She was well-organised too. Despite their different personalities they faced challenges together, running our orchard as a team. When they moved from the farm to Shepparton Mum started work at the local Yakka factory sewing work clothes and ended up managing the place.

I had a relatively positive outlook on life before I became sick. But it did not make sense to say, Yes, I was a positive thinker. I could harbour resentment and regret but rarely had explosions of anger. I did think the best of those I met until they proved otherwise. I had hope that a situation would turn out for the best, with a caveat. Living my comfortable and privileged Australian life sometimes came with powerful lessons. Challenging events happen to all of us of course, often when least expected. However, I generally did not anticipate the worst as my default position.

I see myself as a realist.

I am more wary now. Fears are heightened; I'm more fragile and open to emotional and physical shocks. Current world events make me apprehensive.

The absurdities of life still make me laugh.

Consciously employing positive thinking as a fix-all wellness aid does not gel with me. It generates worries that I cannot meet everyone's expectations or fight the battle. What makes anyone think it will work anyway? Will my mental capacity be up to the task? What if I feel discouraged? Defeated? Is my karma bad? Will I fail to recover and just roll over and die? Tenacity is part of my emotional make-up but I was never interested in beating myself up. I was already on the mat, having experienced high levels of long-term stress through my encounters with the medical system.

After the chemotherapy residual cancer cells still remained in my body. Could mind power stop my chromosomes from making unwanted extra copies? Two doses of targeted, toxic chemicals could not reverse this. Was my mind more powerful in killing cancer cells than chemotherapy? Could my hardworking brain help my cells overcome GVHD? Permanently improve the function of my liver and kidneys? It had not worked yet so for myself, although I wished I could say yes, I had to reluctantly say no, I wasn't a mesmerist. I was not able to control the world with my thoughts.

So in summary I think I am a pragmatic, creative, hard working person who has enjoyed a rewarding and evolving working life and have a supportive husband and community. However it is true that challenging past experiences can have a nasty way of catching up with us and my particular dislike of hospitals and medical procedures would have a direct effect on most aspects of my diagnosis, treatment and ongoing recovery.

TWO

——

Something's wrong

Symptoms appear

In the months preceding the cancer diagnosis I had a sneaking suspicion something was not quite right with my health.

A false start

Towards the end of 2011 the Community Sustainability Program I was running for two rural shires was nearing completion. The free workshops, which offered residents practical information to reduce their energy, water and food bills, avoid waste and create a productive garden, were informative, entertaining and often fully booked. I enjoyed working with my colleagues, presenters and the local community but garnering the energy to make it all happen was becoming more and more difficult. Gardening had always been a passion, and before moving to the country I owned my own horticulture enterprise in Melbourne. Now I could only manage to raise a shovel for a short time before calling it quits. My hair started to thin out. Bruises, sometimes quite large, were appearing for no real reason. A blood vessel burst in my eye, giving me the appearance of someone who had run into a door. The GP told me not to worry about it, that it would heal itself. I was not as interested in food as I normally was. If I scratched myself gardening and licked the cut, my blood did not taste of iron. My energy level could be called one of general low-grade malaise. I thought this must be the way a person felt as they aged. Oddly, I started to ask myself questions about the medical what ifs. What if I had to go to hospital for an operation? How would I cope? I knew the answer to that. Not all that well.

What does Dr Google say?

I had a vague inkling of the worst case scenario. I knew that bruising could indicate leukaemia. There are no screening programs to detect blood cancers. What to do? Look up leukaemia symptoms on Dr Google of course. I ran though the checklist; some of the symptoms matched, one of which was the bruising. When I mentioned this to my colleague Annemaree whose father died after contracting leukaemia she suggested I have my doctor check it out. I spotted the people also ask section on Google. One question stood out – What type of leukaemia is most fatal? Most fatal? Was I going to die soon? Crikey. I think I need an aspirin, a cuppa and a good lie down.

Off to the doctor

I did not talk to anybody, including Fred, about my fears. With what I thought was great courage, I made an appointment with my GP late in 2011. I resigned myself to having a blood test. My regular doctor, whom I only saw infrequently, knew of my life-long, and extreme, needle phobia. Apparently some GPs are not well equipped to deal with blood cancers such as Acute

Myeloid Leukaemia because they do not come across them all that often. As I was to discover, this can delay diagnosis. For AML, a patient should ideally be seen by a haematologist within 24-hours of diagnosis because there is a good reason it is called Acute. When I jokingly suggested that I probably had leukaemia, my doctor thought the bruising was most likely due to the skin getting thinner as I aged. She thought I was in good health generally. I did not make a big deal of my lack of energy or lack of appetite. I was relieved to have avoided the blood test. Nevertheless, I left the clinic feeling a bit cowardly about it. People with needle phobia can be their own worst enemy.

I'm fine – actually I'm not

Three months later illness really kicked in. It started with an even greater level of depleted energy and loss of appetite. My near-neighbour, Sandi, collected me for a wander around Yarra Bend Park. She knew I was having trouble putting one foot in front of the other and asked if I was feeling alright. I'm fine, I replied but I was not fine and she knew it.

Soon I had trouble even leaving the house. The occasional nausea and vomiting now continued day and night for a week. The vomit looked like many little shards of brown glass or coffee grounds which turned out to be blood. I became dehydrated and my energy was totally expended. Somebody call for the doctor, in the immortal words of JJ Cale (and many others). That's what I did. My symptoms were first diagnosed as possible gastro by another GP at the clinic, and then as a possible urinary tract infection (UTI) by a doctor in the Emergency Department at The Alfred Hospital. By this stage I was ready for a blood test; well, not quite ready but reluctantly willing. I asked the Emergency Doctor to test me. He didn't deem it necessary. Due to my needle phobia I was not going to push the point. From memory the Emergency Doctor did a urine test (which tests for white and red blood cells and nitrates). He then gave me a prescription for some tablets for the UTI.

The problem had now been misdiagnosed three times. Walking home from the tram stop after going up the street was misery. I had trouble putting one foot in front of the other and frequently needed to rest. Reaching the flat and putting myself to bed provided little relief. After a fitful nap I awoke feeling just as sick and was losing all interest in food except greasy potato chips.

Finally – four months later – DIAGNOSIS

I wasn't feeling any better in the days that followed. Finally, after visiting my local clinic for a second time in a week (I wasn't seen by my usual doctor but other GPs at the clinic), I had *the* blood test. On 29 March 2012. The phone call came from the doctor at 11.30 pm, just as we were getting ready for bed. My first thought was that this must be serious. I was right. The blood test showed an abnormally high white cell count. The doctor told me I needed to go to the Emergency Department immediately. 'You most likely have leukaemia.'

One sentence. Confirming what I secretly suspected was causing my compromised health. A possible death sentence.

But I reminded myself how modern medicine has altered the Darwinian concept of survival of the fittest. An increased survival rate for many diseases is possible today thanks to our access to excellent medical care. If nature had taken its course I probably would not have lived past childhood, particularly the serious complications from the measles.

There was a chance I might come out of this experience alive.

Despite the Emergency Department doctor previously misreading my symptoms, Melbourne's Alfred Hospital was the only hospital I wanted to be admitted to. The Alfred is an historic institution, founded 150 years ago and named after

Queen Victoria's fourth child, Prince Alfred. It is the second oldest hospital in Victoria, and the oldest still operating at its original site. Even though quite a few of the buildings need updating, The Alfred is a public hospital with a world-wide reputation for a high standard of care. I found that comforting. The staff deal with people needing emergency, intensive and ongoing care – burn cases, accidents, psychiatry, drug overdoses, cystic fibrosis and cardiology, gunshot and knife wounds and of course blood diseases. The entire complex of buildings functions like a mini city, with its own busy café, chemist, newsagent and post office and massive set-up behind the scenes. Fred, his mother Thelma, and several friends, had been treated at The Alfred – everything from kidney stones to HIV and hepatitis C. I had been impressed with the considerate way the hospital staff looked after everyone, especially the palliative care Thelma received after her kidneys failed. Fred, his sister Denise and I stayed overnight in the ward during that time. I remember how surprisingly safe and cocooned I felt. I was not feeling sick myself but thought if I did get ill that night help was immediately at hand.

Help. It's an emergency

The confirmation of leukaemia by the Registrar at The Alfred's Emergency Department came as a big shock on one level, and yet, given the past few months of sluggish health, my symptoms and the doctor's urgent phone call, it did not come as a total surprise. I did not feel positive. I did not feel hopeful.

OK I'll say it – I was probably finished – the end, well and truly stuffed. I was in the gene pool and I was drowning. No more enjoying life with Fred, the man I had spent most of my adult years with, no more being with my mother, family and friends, no more Italian restaurants, no more music or theatre or TV or movies, no more gardening, reading or collecting

Czech art deco pottery. No more travelling overseas, no more fillet steak cooked in butter by my mum as a special treat when I came to visit. No more working to help people live sustainably. Adios and finito!

It was a relief to discover exactly what was ailing me, but oh, how I wished it was only gastro.

I would not have picked myself as a candidate for blood cancer. And there was no history of cancer in my family that I knew of. What did this all mean for me?

THREE

Let the Treatment Begin

Once long ago I did a U-turn right in front of a tram going fast, downhill, in Bourke Street. I was thoroughly told off by a tram worker who happened to be travelling right behind me. Now the cancer tram aimed straight at me and a collision was unavoidable.

Using an image of a yellow rhino on a skateboard, the brilliant 2011 Yarra Trams' *Beware the Rhino* safety campaign emphasised that a tram weighs the equivalent of thirty rhinos. It cannot stop suddenly so it is best not to cross paths with one. I related the rhino images to my cancer experience, especially the cartoon-style yellow and black poster showing a car driver's shocked expression as a tram/rhino was about to crash into their car. That accurately reflected how I perceived my situation.

Hold on. Sudden stops are sometime necessary (due to cancer). Beware. Look. Listen. There will be a service disruption. You never know so don't let go (when you get cancer). In an emergency (get help for cancer). You are being monitored (in hospital). I could go on...

Now I was well and truly on the rhino, sorry, chemotherapy tram. I chose this route, I found myself stuck in the tram

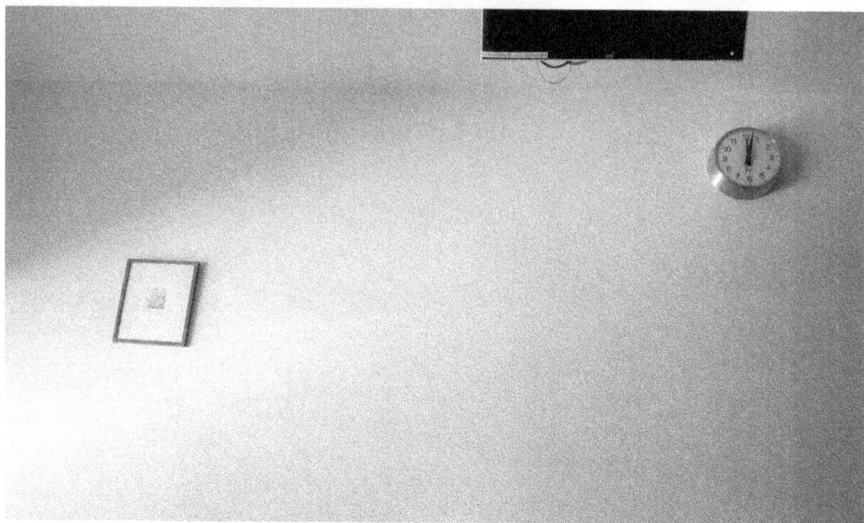

Hospital room – the view from my bed.

tracks and I wasn't getting out of this place anytime soon. Each procedure turned into a kind of mental and physical test and I would feel a modicum of relief and momentary happiness when each was over. The moments between procedures and bouts of nausea would become a haven for me.

The Cancer Card. Playing the hand you are dealt.

The thing I quietly dreaded was happening. I was about to understand that I didn't just have needle phobia but feared the many hospital processes ahead too. I really should have understood this before now. Visits to doctors, when I couldn't avoid them, always made me feel anxious and watching someone else receive an injection made me feel faint. Now I was going into the lion's den 24/7.

What was my treatment regime to be?

I wasn't thinking about alternative treatments. I knew enough about chemotherapy and its potential for severe side effects and no guarantee of a good outcome. What to do? I had a big decision to make. Did I go the chemotherapy route or use the alternative therapy option? Or a combination of both? It was made clear to me by the specialist who had given me my diagnosis that treatment must start immediately. My good friend David had used complementary medicine to treat his prostate cancer and was still alive. I faced certain death without treatment and so I put my faith in the chemotherapy option. I kept my fingers crossed that my body was still strong enough to cope with the toxic chemicals.

My admission to The Alfred Hospital, and the treatment regime that followed, was all about set procedures and systems. It all happened terribly fast. Although I perceived myself to be the first and only person in the world to get cancer, thousands of patients had trodden this path before me. The hospital staff had seen it all before. An identification band was created for my wrist. Every time I had a procedure or received medication or blood products my details were checked, or even double checked by a second nurse, especially when chemotherapy and strong drugs were involved.

Arriving on the ward

Welcome to Ward 7 East, my home for the next month. Upon arrival at the seventh floor turn right for oncology, haematology and stem cell transplants. A large door automatically opened and closed as people came and went. My room was designed for two patients. Luckily at this stage I had the space all to myself. It was the same as many other public hospital rooms, a surprisingly comfortable bed on wheels, sections of which could be manoeuvred up and down, a cupboard, a bedside unit, a washbasin, a holder for recording basic patient details on the wall and another for files at the end of the bed, a rectangular table on wheels which could slide across the top of the bed, an annoying ticking wall clock. Cream walls. A small artwork next to a wall-mounted TV. A row of outlets, holders and sockets for medical equipment, gloves and other accoutrements. A privacy curtain around the bed. You could still hear everything of course. Function won out over style. The space did not have a design aesthetic – it's more a design anaesthetic.

A spacious bathroom conveniently situated next to the room featured linoleum that curved up from the floor to the wall. The room smelled of commercial cleaning products, slightly musty. Outside a row of similar rooms led off a long wide corridor. A nurses' station opposite my room, further along a windowless sitting room with TV and some magazines for patients and guests, a kitchen, offices, staff rooms and storage rooms. A room with a huge bathtub in it. And more sickrooms.

My balcony had a lovely view out to the park. Gardening had been a vital part of my existence. I spent ten years of my working life outdoors in all weathers, but for the next few weeks I would not be going outside, let alone sitting under a tree. Ward 7 East did not have lovely, fresh outside air. The windows did not open, not to stop patients from escaping but to prevent something bad from getting in. The air was twice filtered to reduce the risk of bugs as the patients had low immune systems owing to chemotherapy. A few patients were at such risk of infection that no-one was allowed into their room except for nursing and medical staff. The dried-out processed air reminded me of the atmosphere in an aeroplane; it periodically made me gasp like a redfin thrown on the bank of a river.

Like the rhino on the skate board, the cancer treatment tram was a well-oiled machine moving at full speed ahead but I had no real idea where I was headed. I had my own specialist overseeing my care – Professor David Curtis. He is a clinical haematologist and bone marrow transplant physician and currently oversees a large team as Director of Malignant Haematology Research at the Australian Centre for Blood Diseases, Monash University at The Alfred Hospital.

The Professor's extensive experience inspired confidence. He was there for others and I hoped he was there for me.

Introduction to procedures

I was preoccupied with my perceived inability to cope with all the procedures I had to go through. I decided it was best to look at each one as an obstacle to be faced and then endured. What else could I do? My first day in Ward 7 East on 30 March, was busy. It commenced with a blood test, my second since 1976. I approached it with extreme trepidation, freezing up and holding my breath and praying for it to be over; I was scared stiff. Phew, that's done. Next up was a bone marrow biopsy, the first of five over the coming months. During this procedure local anaesthetic and a sedative were administered, then a bone marrow sample withdrawn via a hollow needle inserted into the back of my right hip. The cells were then examined at the laboratory. In theory this reads like an awful body invasion. In practice quite tolerable thanks to the sedation, and I felt in reasonable spirits afterwards, a temporary rest within the eye of the cyclone. I was reminded of the time I was passenger in a Pan Am Boeing 747 which flew slap bang into a cyclone over Hawaii. The plane rattled, shook, dived and recovered for what seemed like hours. The relief as we entered the quietness of the eye was most welcome. Unfortunately it was followed by another great bout of shaking. When we landed I heard one of the pilots say how impressed he was with the plane's performance. He sounded quite relieved. Lessons learned – it pays to be in the hands of a specialist and even a cyclone has a resting place.

Hickman Line

Next, a visit to the radiology department. Patients in beds were quietly lined up ready for their procedures or tests. Under sterile conditions I lay on my back and my radiologist covered me in cloths. He injected local anaesthetic into the skin in the upper chest then inserted a Hickman catheter into one of the large veins deep inside my chest close to my heart. I will admit to you that I wept and wailed a little bit as he began the procedure. The radiologist kindly waited while I released some tension. Somehow, I could tell he was not going to wait forever. The actual procedure was bearable although I kept my eyes tightly closed the entire time. I distracted myself by noting the Hickman was made of silicone; I had been given a silicone implant but my breast size hadn't changed. The Hickman made the taking of blood and the delivery of drugs and fluids much easier. I viewed it as a precious gift. Not being jabbed with needles was a privilege for anxious patients like me. Still, it felt strange to see tubes coming right out of my chest, anchored by a dressing of transparent adhesive plastic, and I would always feel anxious when the nurse came along to change the dressing. Just in case it was painful.

Heart function

Finally, a test of heart function, also involving needles. Between each procedure I lay there stiffly on my hospital trolley, mostly frozen in terror or numbness, however my mind was racing and my heart going a hundred miles an hour. I was so frightened. I feared being hurt. Jabbed and cut and prodded. Somewhere from within me I called on my meagre reserves of courage to cope with what was being done to me. I experienced tremendous relief as each procedure was completed and I counted the hours until the whole thing was over for the day. At times my natural inclination for curiosity kicked in. I amused myself and passed the time by observing exactly how the hospital functioned. The initial impression? Non-stop activity.

After all this I could not wait to eat the delicious noodles in clear soup brought by my girlfriend Duré from her restaurant. My family – my mother, my brothers Peter and John and nieces Danielle and Stephanie – paid a visit. I was bouncing around on the bed in party mode, driven by the adrenalin rush of surviving my first day. I somehow managed to deal with my intense fear of needles and medical procedures. My mum said, 'I know you are sick but you don't look it.' That was because I was a hero who had survived day one of the so-called cancer journey. I could recall many more enjoyable trips. I had faced my worst medical demons and coped with horrifying procedures all day long, plus being topped up with rehydrating fluids. Actually, I was in shock. Everyone I knew and loved was stunned too. I was healthy before this. I felt sure some people were thinking, If it could happen to Cathy...

Communications – who and how to tell

Fred and I spent the evening asking each other how the hell did this happen and decided on how to manage communications with family and friends.

I made two big decisions to help me survive the next few weeks. The AML was not to be kept a secret. I was not ashamed to have cancer, I happened to have cancer, like millions of people around the planet, so what was the point. (According to BBC.com someone in the world is diagnosed with blood cancer every 35 seconds. AML is relatively rare; around 1,100 Australians are diagnosed each year with the disease. Although the median age at diagnosis is around sixty-five, AML affects young people too.) Keeping it quiet would use far too much energy and it was difficult to do when you have lost your hair and can't walk properly. And a public hospital was not the best place to hide out anyway. I already happened to know two people who work at The Alfred, one of them a senior nurse.

Although I was happy to advertise my AML to the world, my friend Paulette pointed out that every patient is entitled to privacy. It was not the right of others to broadcast details of a person's illness if they don't want anyone to know. There were strong arguments for not telling. It depended on each person's situation. Did you tell young children? Were you famous and didn't want your business discussed on the front page of a trashy magazine? Would the boss sack you? Discrimination by employers who feared the disease would return is a real issue. I did not have a job to go to (and did not mention my illness when I later attended job interviews).

No visitors

After the initial visits, I decided virtually no visitors except Fred until I was better able to cope with the treatment and its side effects.

Now I am recovered and feeling reasonably well I look back and wish I had not done this. At the time I couldn't do anything else. I did not have the resources to answer anyone's questions or have a chat. Even sending a text message was a huge task taking all my strength.

Having a room full of visitors may be some patient's idea of heaven. It was my idea of a nightmare. I could not bear the thought of being asked to explain how I was feeling. I found it taxing enough to meet the demands of the hospital routine. If you are in a shared ward, healthy visitors surrounding the next bed often party and chat. They can forget why we are here. Quiet everyone. We are trying to be sick here and might even be dying. Being nauseous or in pain, you may not need to hear all about their fun weekend jet-skiing, Aunty Alice dropping in for a cup of tea or what Junior did or did not do at play school.

Leukaemia – how does it work?

As I mentioned, the particular leukaemia I had is Acute Myeloid Leukaemia. Acute is far worse than chronic, as the name suggests, and treatment needs to commence immediately as the disease progresses quickly. If you are dealing with blood cancer it is not essential to be an information maven, but over time I found it helpful to grasp exactly what was happening inside my body. Some patients are naturally science oriented. They love to study up. They want to understand every aspect of their disease. When I was first admitted to hospital the only thing I knew about leukaemia was that it was a disease of the blood and could cause bruising, lethargy and loss of appetite. That's it. I'm getting ahead of myself, but in the early weeks of treatment my brain shut down in the knowledge department. I couldn't tell the difference between platelets, neutrophils and blast cells. To take charge of your own treatment to some extent you do need to know what has happened inside your body. My understanding of AML took some years.
Here is what I learned:

It is all about our cells and what is inside them. Our bodies are so incredible. All human cells must start with DNA; it contains the code to tell each cell how to initially construct itself. The nucleus is the cell's command centre. Inside these nuclei are twenty-three pairs of chromosomes. These are tightly wound strings made up of DNA which look like a twisted ladder – a double helix. More than two metres of DNA is inside every single one of these cells; a tightly packed setup, with each chromosome containing one DNA molecule. This DNA, which is made up of genes, contains the instructions an organism needs to develop, function and reproduce. It is my unique generic code, half inherited from my mother and the other half from my father. Around 25,000 genes determine my physical traits and give my cells orders as to the type of cell it will become, how to behave, and when to multiply or give up the ghost. All my blood cells originate from stem cells which are made in bone marrow, the spongy part in the centre of my bones. Early on, they develop into either myeloid stem cells (red blood cells, platelets and all white blood cells apart from lymphocytes) or lymphoid stem cells (white blood cells called lymphocytes). Diseases of the blood cells, like leukaemia, can cause this balance to be thrown out. There are more than forty unique sub-types of leukaemia. AML, which is not just a single disease, is a leukaemia of the white blood cells that develops in the myeloid cell line in the bone marrow.

The main symptoms of AML include: anaemia, and easy bleeding and/or bruising due to inadequate numbers of red cells and platelets being made by the bone marrow; persistent tiredness; dizziness, paleness, or shortness of breath when physically active and frequent or repeated infections and slow healing, due to a lack of normal white cells, especially neutrophils. Other symptoms may include bone pain, swollen lymph nodes, swollen gums, chest pain and abdominal discomfort due to a swollen spleen or liver. The only outward symptoms I had which matched this list were tiredness and bruising. As for the inside...

I have a photograph of myself taken two weeks before my diagnosis. To me it is an image of a sickly-looking woman who still happened to be walking around. My skin had a yellow pallor which indicated liver trouble, the whites of my eyes were grey and I exuded tiredness. And no wonder. A normal white cell count is 10-11 x 109/L while my count was 43 x 109/L! And all of those cells were of the useless, immature kind.

There are billions of cells inside our bodies. It is so easy to take these cells for granted until something goes wrong. When the body is healthy, the numbers of red cells (which do not have a nucleus), white cells and platelets in the blood are kept in balance. Each time a cell divides into two new cells, it must make a new copy of its chromosomes. Mistakes can happen when cells divide. These mutations are usually repaired, or if the cells are badly damaged the immune system may see them as abnormal and eliminate them. My body had been efficiently attacking any faulty cells or unwanted invaders for fifty-nine years; quite a long time. Now something had gone awry on the production line of my cell-making factory. A mistake had been made in copying the genetic material and the workers had created the wrong type of cell. An overproduction of immature white blood cells, called myeloblasts or leukaemic blasts, had overwhelmed my bone marrow, preventing it from making normal blood cells. Because of their immaturity,

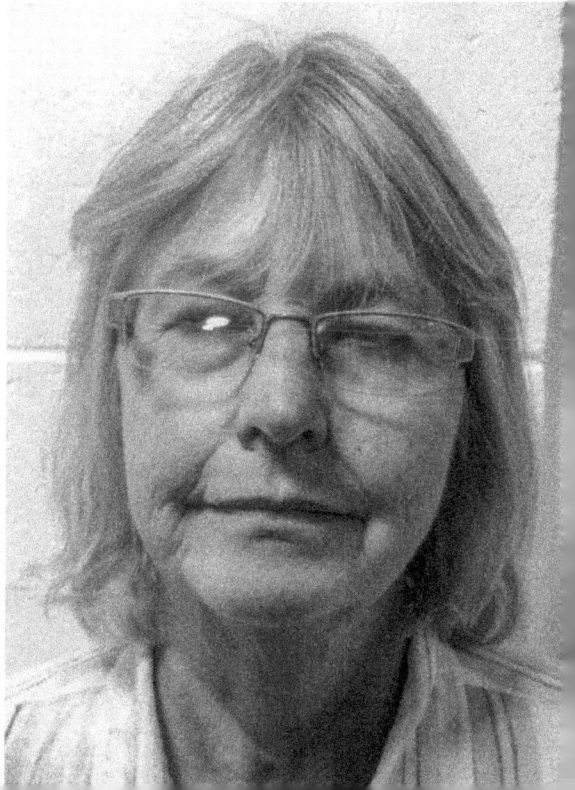

12 March 2012.

they were unable to function properly to prevent or fight infection. Normal cells did not have any room to grow in the bone marrow and these leukaemia cells took over the normal function of the bone marrow.

Why were so many dud white cells being produced? With leukaemia, chromosomes join together or mutate. Genetic changes found in AML include: chromosomes undergoing a translocation, which means that big chunks of the DNA rearrange themselves; a chromosome breaks off and reattaches to another chromosome; inversions occur when part of a chromosome gets turned around; an extra copy is made or a chromosome is deleted.

Leukaemia cells are clever. I admit to a sneaking admiration of their tricky ability to avoid being killed off. Even though the body is constantly recognising and mopping up the clones of abnormal cells, somehow these cells are able to evade this protective mechanism by producing a don't-eat-me signal making the body unable to recognise the error and correct it.

The most important factor in predicting my chances of a cure was the genetic make-up of these leukaemic cells. The science is complex but the profile of my AML read like this: trisomies 8.21; FLT3, NPM1, TKD [mutations] all negative. For some reason my body made an extra copy of chromosomes 8 and 21 instead of the usual pair. An extra chromosome 8 is not unusual in AML, but less so an extra chromosome 21. And two extras are seen less frequently than one extra. This indicated an average prognosis; my chances of recovery were not great but it was not the worst-case scenario either.

Chemotherapy starts

Counter-intuitively, chemotherapy reduces the ability of the bone marrow to produce adequate numbers of blood cells and platelets. I was told my blood counts would fall within a week of treatment and may take some time to recover, depending on the type and doses of drugs my doctor decided on. During this time I would be given antibiotics and other drugs to treat, or prevent infection, along with blood transfusions to treat severe anaemia, and platelet transfusions to reduce the risk of bleeding. I had some challenging side effects to look forward to. Chemotherapy affects rapidly growing normal, healthy cells such as hair follicles as well as cancer cells. Other possible side-effects include: feeling sick – nausea and/or vomiting, feeling fatigued and weak, hair loss and thinning, mouth problems such as mucositis or ulcers, diarrhoea or constipation, skin problems such as dryness, rash or sensitivity to sunlight. Bring it on!

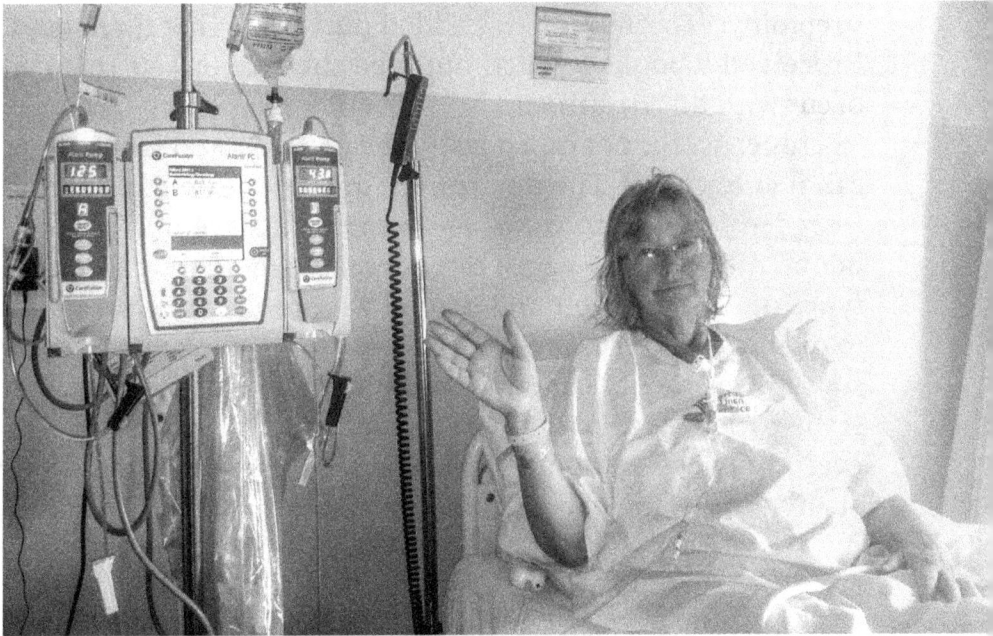

Day two of chemo, 31 March 2012.

There is a Dutch saying Mum liked to use when setting my hair in tight plastic curlers. Wie mooi wil zijn, moet pijn lijden. The English translation: If you want to be beautiful, you have to endure pain.

Life-threatening diseases such as AML have their price as well. Chemotherapy is without doubt a brutal regime. And if I wanted to pursue the possibility of a cure I had to endure pain. Otherwise death was inevitable within weeks or months or maybe even days. That was my immediate non-negotiable future.

No time was wasted at cancer central. On the second day of admittance chemotherapy commenced. I was given Cytarabine by drip into the vein for seven days continuously. According to Cancer Research UK, anti-metabolites such as Cytarabine are similar to normal body molecules but they are slightly different in structure. They kill cancer cells by stopping them making and repairing DNA that they need to grow and multiply. A top up of fifteen minutes of Idarubicin (a drug extracted from streptomyces bacterium) was added during the first three days. I received a booklet which outlined the side effects that can occur with this treatment.

This cancer is not called acute for nothing. And I would not call it cute either. The doctors and nurses told me only what I needed to know to move on to the next stage of treatment but no more. At this stage I did not realise there were different types of AML or even understood what leukaemia was doing to my body. I later asked Paulette what her approach was at the start of treatment. She told me she was guided by the patient. If the patient desired information she might say, I can tell you everything we are doing today and why. Please ask questions at any time. If the patient chose to be silent, that was OK too.

I'm scared – again

I felt afraid, very afraid. An all-encompassing feeling. Scared of lying alone in my hospital bed. Afraid of what the future held. Afraid I wouldn't have the courage to face the next procedure. I did not feel like crying. I didn't tremble. I did not try to flee or fight. I simply went stiff and held my breath most of the time.

We are called patients for a reason – because utmost patience is required. Every day in hospital, (and the days at home between treatments), was a test of fortitude and boredom often set in. There was not much point in thinking too much about the future as it could be a waste of energy. At this moment I needed to comply with the system and deal with the substantial side effects of the chemo, not use energy pushing impotently against the whole experience before I knew what I was pushing against.

Make your space your own

Some tips for anyone being admitted to the cancer ward – pimp up your bed and while you are at it buy some nice pyjamas and dressing gown. You are going to be using this bed for quite some time. It will become your sanctuary, your oasis. The nurses put a plastic sheet underneath the bottom bedsheet for obvious reasons. Grab one of the cotton blankets provided and put it under the bedsheet. No more sliding around and down the bed, much cosier. I brought my own down-filled pillow and wore colourful woollen bed socks knitted by Mum. Add to this a sheepskin rug from mates Ronda and Tim and pricey triple-milled Italian soap and I was good to go. And I had twenty-four-hour room service for food, fluids and drugs. Plus a buzzer for assistance. Nearly as smart as a hotel. I had staff!

When you remove the little clip from your finger which monitors heart-rate, or turn over and unsettle the intravenous drip, the machine will make an annoying non-stop buzzing or continuous beeping noise. Over time you will figure out how

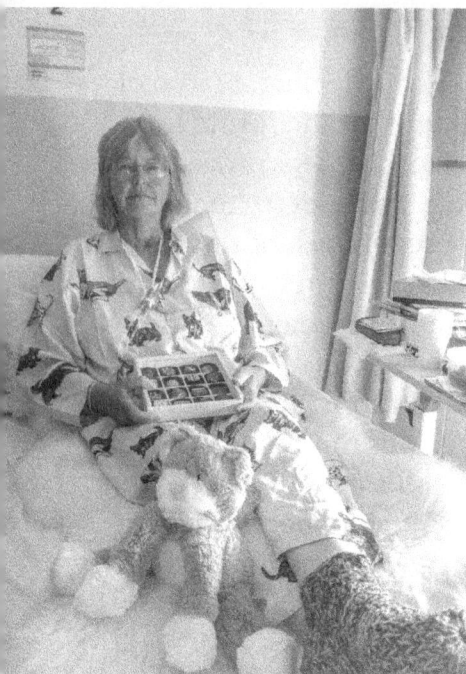

Third day of chemo, 1 April 2012.

to adjust the machine yourself, however that is a job best left to the nurses. You can also check the chart pocketed at the end of the bed. It makes for exciting reading if you are into numbers. And you will need to be.

If you love to read like I do, chemo brain may mean a small magazine article is all you can manage. Reading a book from cover to cover required far too much concentration. Even the usual stuff on TV was difficult to watch. Some people are said to have a mind like a steel trap. During chemo my mind was more like a rusty tin lid.

Having a shower

The chemo had taken away my usual body aromas. I hardly sweated, didn't smell strongly and didn't have a good sense of smell or taste either. It seemed like these senses had chemically been stripped from me in a systematic fashion, layer by layer. In regards to bathing, I love to be clean (and confess I rinse the soap before and after I use it). Getting back into the hospital bed after a shower was the best feeling in the world. Showering in a medical situation involved some tricky manoeuvres. The nurse detached me from the tubes and covered the Hickman with water-proof plastic, yet I still feared the water would get into my heart and kill me. I was relieved when I emerged from the bathroom unscathed. Going to the toilet was fun too when the medical equipment and metal stand on wheels had to accompany me. Taking a tee-shirt off with all the paraphernalia attached was a challenge and occasionally it ended up being cut off. It was a great relief when the drip was finally removed after the first week of chemo.

So much waste!

If you are into recycling it can be a shock to see how much medical waste is generated due to potential contamination issues and perceived lower cost of single-use items. While having the Hickman port cleaned, I noted how each piece of material in the sterile kit was used once, or not used at all, and then folded up and thrown away.

According to The Alfred's Facebook page from August 2019:

> *Every year, we go through more than 140,000 single-use metal instruments like scissors, scalpels and tweezers – which are currently sent to landfill. But as part of an exciting pilot program to drastically reduce how much waste we produce, we're looking at recycling these stainless steel instruments – which can be melted down and re-used.*

I wondered how many instruments were sterilised and reused, like they used to do in the old days. On another positive note, providing patients with water from a jug meant many single-use plastic bottles of water were not being consumed.

The day started early

I dictated my day to Fred so he could send an email to everyone. Hospitals are not the place to relax and kick back. A great deal of work goes into treating you and then making sure the side effects of treatment are reduced. One aspect I did not comment on was how rarely medical staff seemed to interact with the cleaners or food and drink deliverers. Sometimes it was like they were working in parallel universes.

Midnight	Observations (obs.) by the nurse – heart rate and oxygenation, blood pressure, temperature.
	Half asleep.
4.00am	Repeat above but this time blood taken from ye olde port in my chest. Hickman's Port or some other name – we call it Hicksville (and call chemo Drano, no offense to the product).
7.00am	I wake up nauseous.
	Anti-nausea drugs delivered via Hickman. Fill out food order for next day.
8.00am	Breakfast, including fruit in syrup for cereal imported from China. What are they thinking? Why not use local Goulburn Valley fruit?
	Description of breakfast – hideous.
	Room cleaning starts, water person does water jugs, rubbish person collects rubbish.
	I jokingly refer to all the people – there must be over twenty-five – as my staff.
	Tablets taken.
	Anti-fungal mouth wash (many times a day).
	Anti-thrush liquid etc.
	Another round of obs. taken.
	Time to be weighed (in a weighing chair) to check fluid retention issues. Tricky balance of fluid balancing act – so diuretics are regularly given, leading to needing to go to the toilet every 5 minutes – boring.
9.00am	Doctor arrives with pile of students in tow – five

of them. Students do routine stuff under direction from boss.

10am	First blood transfusion set up and delivered via Hickman plus some other drugs.
	Time for a shower done by nurse. No repeat of the earlier Fred debacle where he sprayed more water on himself than on the patient.
11am	Priest comes in and asks if he can say some prayers over me.
12.00pm	Next set of observations.
	Lunch quite nice – falafels.
	This is a big day – with two sachets of blood delivered. I feel guilty not ever having given blood, now someone else is saving my life!
1.00pm	Social worker arrives for a bit of therapy (me, not social worker – I don't feel I need their help, I have Fred).
2.00pm	Visit from the plasma people to discuss bone marrow donor possibilities. Whilst the plasma has been delivered obs. are taken every 15 minutes to check reactions.
3.00pm	Nurses deliver more oral medications. (Always given in a little plastic cup).
4.00pm	Next set of obs.
4.15pm	Read a magazine.
5.00pm	Dinner arrives – eat soup.
	More diuretics pumped in.
5.30pm	Fred arrives with new PJs, undies, laptop computer, latest emails etc.
8.00pm	More obs.
10.00pm	Sleeping pill taken.

| 10.30pm | Fred leaves. |
| Midnight | Obs. taken – off on another day of action. |

There is another thing I should have added to this list. The nurses regularly asked, Do you have any pain? and Would you like a Panadol? I did consider asking for some morphine. As you can see chemo brain was already kicking in. I was curious to experience the effect of morphine, in theory anyway. Not pleasant from what Mum told me.

Regarding the fruit imported from China, our orchard near Shepparton produced peaches, pears and apricots. I asked the patient liaison officer to put in a complaint to management with a request that they only provide Australian fruit. You don't run a sustainability program for three years without learning something about food miles, cost saving and dodgy food quality in far-off lands.

More presents

The gifts kept coming – cards with loving messages, fruit such as rockmelon beautifully shaped like real flowers, beanies, pyjamas, an MP3 player, a DVD on meditation techniques, a lovely book by country chef Annie Smithers, a grey cat soft toy, a hand spun and hand knitted scarf and hat from an ex-colleague at the shire, along with emailed photos of a newly born baby, a black cow called Milky, lovely landscapes and gardens and a Gould's Long-eared bat. Dr Russ Harris, the bestselling author of *The Happiness Trap* and a long-term friend, dropped in with a copy of his latest book, *The Reality Slap: How to Find Fulfilment When Life Hurts*. I didn't tell Russ until later that it was gathered up in the bed sheets and probably ended up in the hospital laundry. Hopefully it did not make a mess of their industrial washing machine.

No more takeaways

Once the chemo took effect, food could not be brought in from outside. My neutrophils, a type of abundant white blood cell, were now low (this is called neutropenia). As a consequence my immune system could not easily fight bacteria or viruses that cause infections, as I was to find out in dramatic fashion later on. Raw or under-cooked meat such as sushi or salami, raw eggs, unpasteurised milk and cheese, pates, shellfish, soft-whip ice cream and unwrapped food such as salads were now forbidden.

Putting on weight rather than losing weight would become a key focus; a matter of survival of the fattest.

Here's a sample of the food on offer. It all came on a large tray and naturally I ate in bed.

Breakfast	I chose cereal with full cream milk, a slice of white bread with vegemite, teabag tea. Plain but edible.
Lunch	A salad of lettuce, tomato and tuna. Plain but fresh.
Dinner	Vegetable soup, roast beef with gravy, boiled carrots, beans and roast potatoes, custard, an orange, apple juice. Just plain. The roast was covered in a maroon-coloured dome of heavy plastic which kept it warm. I couldn't eat the entire dish; the meat was edible but, except for the potatoes, the vegies needed butter, herbs and spices for added flavour.

I didn't expect the hospital food to be five star but visual appeal, freshness and flavour are important to patients undergoing chemo, theoretically anyway. At this stage it didn't matter what was put in front of me. My appetite had almost disappeared and many foods I normally took pleasure in repulsed me. I love Italian food but if you had put the most delicious home-made lasagne in front of me at that moment I would not finish it. I couldn't eat the gorgeous box of chocolates I was given, or enjoy a strong latte, because the chemo had totally altered the way food tasted. Baby foods were what I wanted. Jellies, custards, white toast with vegemite, baked beans, milk, smoothies and two-fruits. And what about alcohol? Before illness struck I drank at most two glasses of white wine with dinner and often did not drink from one day to the next, so it was not something I missed.

Reflections of the bedridden

So what exactly was I feeling and thinking as I lay in my fancied-up hospital bed day after day with tubes attached? Tiredness and fatigue were my constant companions. Sometimes I felt down. Really down. When this happened I didn't want to get up out of bed. Using the bathroom took a huge effort. It could not be put off and I certainly didn't want the nurses to change the bed sheets unnecessarily. I accepted I was joined to a weird mechanical growth. I had learned to manoeuvre into the bathroom, taking care not to bump my beloved Hickman.

Dealing with waves of nausea was not easy either. When the sick feeling came I did not try to hold it down; it was a losing proposition. I picked up the long plastic bag lying on the bedside table, opened up my chest and throat and let the vomit rise. I was amazed at how fast it shot out and I enjoyed the feeling of relief that came afterwards.

Waves of melancholia occasionally overwhelmed me, but I did not tell the nurses. I looked for distractions, yet I couldn't concentrate on any one thing for long. I didn't want to sit up. I didn't feel like watching TV at all now. I tried to escape into sleep, but it often didn't work. Thoughts tumbled in my head one after the other. I had become frightened in a whole new way. I had not faced the possibility of my own demise before this time. I had turned tail and retreated into an emotional limbo. I had gone into my shell. Come and get me. Reach me if you can. At these moments I had given up hope.

I counted the minutes until Fred arrived. When he walked in the door, often with copies of loving emails sent by family and friends, the world felt like a better place again. We caught up on the day's events, we took a slow walk up and down the corridor and I scored a blissful foot massage. We hung out until it was time for him to leave. I missed my own bed and I missed Gus sleeping on my lap but didn't dwell on it too much. It wasn't going to happen anytime soon.

I accepted there was a good chance I might die.

Fortunately, I could say anything to Fred without him judging me or saying, get over yourself, stop it, don't feel bad or put on a happy face. If I needed to cry, I cried. And I did not cry at all in this early stage of treatment. I had gone to a place beyond tears. Although encouraged when the doctors or nurses came around with positive news, much of the time I was simply dazed and confused.

I used a particular technique which made it easier to cope with stress. I had positive thoughts, some of them fleeting, yet I tried to accept the extreme feelings of anxiety as they surfaced. I subscribe to the idea that the more I face up to my apprehension, fear, and loss, I have a greater chance of experiencing the positive emotions too. I can't deny the bad feelings and pushing them down is ultimately counter-productive. They are scary but just as important as the positive feelings. In hospital I told myself I could cope with these feelings; I knew from past experience that they were not going to kill me; my circumstances would change and I had to find a way through. Feelings of worry and confusion can sometimes pass quite quickly if you let them in. The key was to accept all the emotions jostling inside me, positive or negative, cheerful or downcast; an approach I have tried to follow throughout my adult life. I don't see feelings as necessarily bad or good, they just are and they keep changing. It is important to express these emotions or at least recognize them, rather than struggle unsuccessfully to bottle them up. And if my negative thoughts were going round my head like a stuck record and were magnified through being in hospital, I deliberately tried to steer them in a new direction and replace them with more upbeat thoughts. That did make me feel a bit better about the world.

Blood tests were done every day. The aim of the chemo was to wipe out the components such as the white and red cells, platelets and neutrophils and build them up again, hopefully with the cancer cells being wiped out in the process. The nurses recorded the numbers on a sheet of paper. As an example, haemoglobin was 136 on admission on 29 March and down to 96 on 19 April, white blood cells 41 down to 1.1, platelets 80 to 26 and neutrophils 5.74 to 0.04. As noted earlier, during this phase you are highly susceptible to infections. I'm not quite sure how anyone receiving chemo still has the ability to function at all given these low blood levels. One of the nurses commented on the marvellous way our bodies can recover after chemo. Her significant words stayed with me.

Give me a head without hair

I had to face losing my hair. Women are not supposed to be confident about their looks as that would lead to a severe drop in sales for beauty products and reduced demand for plastic surgery but I did have thick, lustrous, dark blonde hair once. Most women are understandably distressed at having their locks fall out by the handful. I was beyond caring about it. However, it was not pleasant having the strands of hair collect in my comb. So rather than wait to go bald, Fred shaved the

whole shebang off for me with
electric clippers. I did not like
looking at myself in the mirror.
Still, everyone told me my head
shape suited being bald. I guess
that was a compliment. I took
another look and saw a more than
passing resemblance to my father.
I never contemplated wearing a
wig. Far too much hassle and far
too hot, like a mini heater on the
head. Welcome gifts of hats rolled
in, include hand knits (one made
from home-spun wool), another of
Harris Tweed and a purple beanie
depicting a mouse complete with
an embroidered face and ears on
top. I wore them in bed.

15 April 2012.

Scalp hypothermia, a treatment which can reduce hair loss,
was introduced to Australia in 2012. A silicone cap is filled
with liquid which is pumped through the cap at a cold 4°C.
The cap is worn for half an hour before chemo and at least
an hour afterwards. I preferred a bald head to a freezing cold
scalp accompanied by a brain freeze, especially as my brain
had already frozen from the chemo.

My eyebrows and eyelashes were the only hairy parts I had
left anywhere on my body. One of the nurses had a laugh
with me about lack of hair in other places while she gave me a
welcome wash. I said, 'I certainly don't need a Brazilian wax!'
We talked about the trend of being hairless down below (for
men and women) and how boyfriends nowadays seemed to
like and even demand it, which made me muse on the pressure
on young women to look pre-pubescent. Or like a porn star?

Let's face it; any talk about feeling (or being) sexy in hospital
(and during convalescence) is more academic than actual for

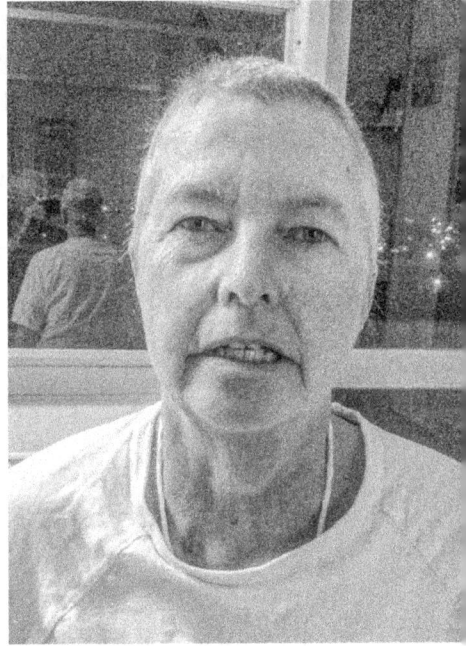

most cancer patients. What with the nausea, vomiting, blood tests, chemo brain, IV drip, tablet taking to counteract the chemo side effects and people coming in and out of the room every five minutes...

Over the next few months my hair (on my head) grew back thick and somewhat curly. I stopped using hair dyes and tried to embrace my new hair colour – a few shades of grey. For some reason my eyebrows and lashes remained dark brown.

First taste of freedom

Alfred Central is a serious place but amusing events can happen there too. Occasionally patients can't take any more and make good an escape. I thought of going AWOL myself at times but, unlike many other patients, did not want to be seen in the hospital foyer in my flannelette pyjamas and furry slippers. I heard about one woman who exited the building without approval and jumped on the No. 72 tram to the city, pastel hospital gown neatly tied up at the back, beeping IV apparatus and all.

Leaving hospital (with permission and without my IV drip) after the first induction round of chemotherapy felt weird. I had been on a cocktail of tablets in the ward and Fred and I now waited for the hospital pharmacist to stock up my home supply. He asked me if I had any allergies, I answered no, he gave me a truckload of drugs in a big plastic bag, a sort of medical doggie bag, and a handy tablet container with a separate removable compartment for each day of the week. I told him there wouldn't be any space left in my stomach for food after I took all these tablets.

I was now outside. Everything struck me as surreal and spaced out, from the footpath to the trees and nearby buildings. The distance between objects was all wrong, like when I accidentally smoked that joint which had horse tranquiliser added many years before. I couldn't walk well. I was not myself at all. My brain had become foggy. It was like being underwater fully kitted out with diving gear. Luckily Fred was driving me home to our flat at Xavier College.

Because a low-level bacterial infection had developed, a pump was attached to my Hickman line. It was cleverly programmed to automatically delivery antibiotics every few hours. I worried, unnecessarily, that it wouldn't work properly. A Hospital-in-the-Home nurse came to the flat daily to change dressings and do observations. After spending two weeks in hospital, my energy levels were at a low ebb. I didn't feel like doing anything, just sitting on the couch wearing a woollen hat and watching a bit of TV while Gus slept contentedly on my lap.

I could now finally entertain visitors, including my mother.

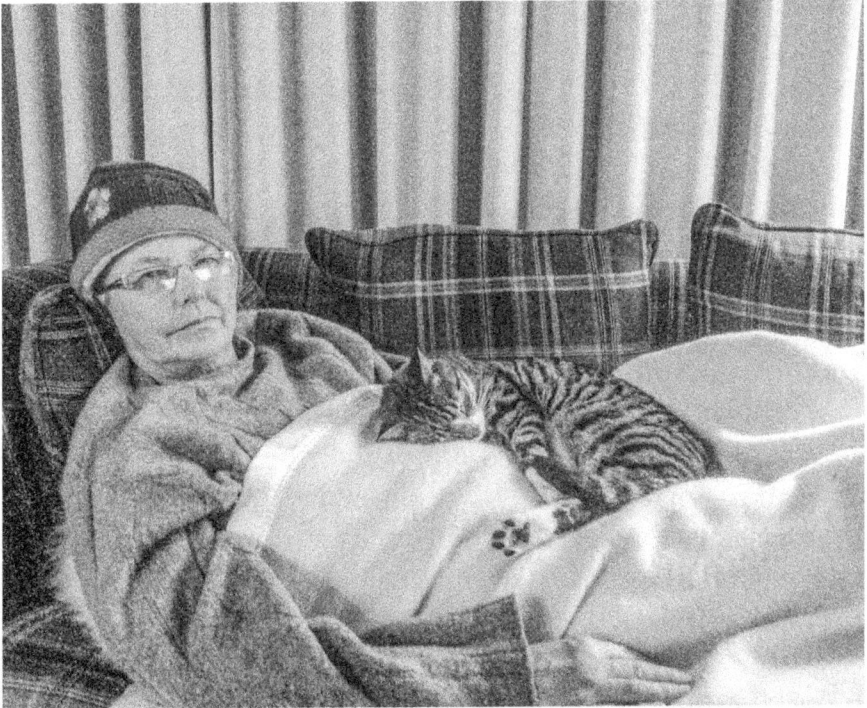

Back at the flat, 3 May 2012.

Sandi brought over a delicious gourmet lunch of gravlax. I ate it and promptly threw up. She wasn't offended. Fred convinced me a walk would do some good. While I didn't want to walk anywhere except to the fridge, the bed or the bathroom I agreed. We did a slow circuit around the boarding house gardens and outside in the well-tended school grounds. Fred helped me negotiate the stairs of the chapel and we sat looking out towards the city. As the sun went down the skyscrapers in the distance were bathed in a soft orange glow. He was pleased to have me home and I was happy to be home.

I could barely make it back to the flat.

Outpatient

My status at The Alfred now changed from inpatient to outpatient. Sometimes Fred drove me to hospital appointments but often I took my weary bones for a trip on the thirty-tonne rhino. It was exhausting to walk to the tram stop when all I yearned for was to sit down. Depending on the day and the results of my blood test, I might be up for a blood transfusion, platelets or magnesium infusion or on special days a bone marrow biopsy.

The Outpatient Department was a busy place. In a room called the Transit Lounge there were cancer patients sitting in oversized chairs with wide arms, their own arms outstretched and tubes draping from Hickmans, PICC lines and cannulas, like a row of dairy cows being milked. Some patients were put on a drip to take the blood out of their bodies. That seemed strange to me, until it was explained their iron levels had become elevated due to the numerous transfusions. As a result, some blood needed to be removed but it wouldn't be suitable for transfusions.

On one of these visits I triggered an emergency code blue. I looked around at all the other patients sitting in their chairs with tubes hanging from their bodies; I unexpectedly became overwhelmed and promptly fainted. Although it was a relief to pass out it did not last anywhere near long enough, just a few seconds. I told the assembled doctors and nurses I was alright but the nurse still needed to do an electrocardiograph to check heart function. She covered my chest in stickers with metal knobs in the centre and yes, my heart was fine.

Outpatient visits demand a very patient demeanour. You can spend hours and hours in the chair. One day I spent half a day there waiting for the Registrar to decide on the next course of action – magnesium or no magnesium infusion. It is easy to get angry in these situations. My advice is to stay calm and carry on. The staff are doing their best dealing with their own not-insubstantial pressures and long work hours. I retreated to my place of Zen, my place of meditation. My place of checking out all the comings and goings; I pretended I was in the audience watching an exciting new play or medical drama. Except nothing much exciting was happening. When the Registrar did finally turn up I was quite pleased to see her.

Second round of chemotherapy

Having built up some strength and with my earlier infection cleared up with antibiotics and rest, I needed to return to The Alfred for a consolidating round of chemotherapy; one kind of strong chemo material to be delivered every two days for a week. The doctors said no sign of AML were found in the previous, albeit meagre, bone marrow sample and they felt I was now in remission and should be in the ward for about ten days. This was standard procedure. Although I did not feel ready for the next onslaught I was told it was better not to leave it too long after the first chemo. I hoped I would have time to build up my blood counts further. It reminded me of being in a boxing ring or those blow up dolls that bounce right back after being punched. I had to be knocked out and get up again. My plans for daily visits to my favourite coffee shops and lying around in my PJs like the Queen of Sheba receiving more visitors were now changed.

I was feeling perky at this moment and ready for the next and hopefully final chemo round. For no good reason at times I thought I would survive. I didn't see myself as brave – I carried on like a big sook when I had some procedures – but so far, I had kept a strong sense of humour/absurdity and had connected well with the hospital staff which certainly helped. I had a strange sort of disease – it affected my entire body yet my heart and other organs were working well. However, unlike a cancerous tumour, it couldn't be operated on because blood is a tissue with many different functions. You can't cut out leukaemia like you can a lump in the breast. It is not an organ with a specific job to do. And it is not totally liquid. I learned blood is over half liquid which is made up of plasma, and half solids such as red cells, white cells and platelets.

The advantage this time around was that I understood what to expect of the hospital routine and the possible side effects of nausea and lack of appetite. I planned to bring in more of my own food (and speculated if my little protest against foreign two fruits had any affect) and spending more time fantasising how to buck the hospital routine. I contemplated telling the nurses I'd become a Jehovah Witness like Prince and couldn't receive any more red blood and plasma. Maybe not such a good idea!

Scars

Around this time I discovered an odd side effect of chemo – the heightened prominence of childhood scars. I had one on my knee where I hit the road after my beach bag became caught in the front wheel of my bike. A second scar resulted from a botched attempt to swing standing up, no hands. I must have been a circus performer in another life. I inevitably lost my balance, fell flat on my face and my top teeth bit right through underneath my bottom lip. The scar from when a metal sprinkler head hit me above the eye as a three-year-old did not reappear and the small dog bite scar across my nose did not change.

The hospital routine continued.

I emailed an update before I returned to the ward and Fred sent another seven days later. Keeping everyone in the loop was now routine.

During my second admission the relationship between patients and nurses found me ruminating. The nurses came from many different countries – Australia, India, the Philippines, South Africa and Ireland. I gravitated to those who were relaxed and friendly; others had a more mechanical and businesslike approach to the work which left me feeling like I was being processed. A few had a bossy or grumpy edge to them. One had lost the tip of a finger in a losing tussle against a lawn mower blade. Some had tattoos which I liked to check out. Because of the Florence Nightingale type of work they do, it is easy to see them as saintly, but to use a cliché; they are human like the rest of us with their own dramas and problems.

Each morning, usually after breakfast, the Professor and his entourage dropped by to receive the progress report from the nurses. Of necessity everybody talked as if I was not there. I found myself wanting to interrupt and offer details such as – My platelets have improved slightly since yesterday or The oxygenation saturation level is 99%. But I didn't. Instead I liked to check out the clothing they were all wearing. I noted the Professor's crisp striped shirt and new trousers; the freshly washed cotton shirts, name tags, the smell of deodorant, the shoes of the female staff which ranged from high heels for some interns to comfortable flats for the nurses. Nurses regularly came up close to the bed, leaning over me to do the obs. I checked what they wore too.

Staying alert must present a challenge for nursing staff who work the night shift. Sometimes the workplace became tense. I was not eavesdropping but I overheard one nurse having an issue with her colleague who had forgotten a procedure. Oops. Maybe these comments about mistakes shouldn't be made within the hearing of patients.

There is one aspect of being a patient which I liked and appreciated. I had absolutely no responsibility for anything, except getting up and going to the toilet once in a while, forcing a morsel of food down, answering Professor Curtis's questions when he came on his rounds and being awake when Fred came to visit. Although I would never fake illness such as Munchausen syndrome or intentionally make myself sick, I understood the attraction of being looked after in hospital. I did not have to hunt for a new job, go shopping, pay bills and taxes or feed the cat or even feed myself. Every time I commented that my treatment must be costing a small fortune, the nurses said, 'Don't worry about that. Just concentrate on getting well.' So I did. The world revolved around me. I was sitting pretty, a passive clown in clover. Then something happened which I didn't like.

Infection

Blood was taken from the Hickman early each morning. Because the chemotherapy reduced the level of white and red bloods cells and made me more susceptible to infections, my temperature was constantly monitored. Signs of a fever were taken seriously. Urgent action was required if it hit 38°C and above. As is commonly the case with cancer patients, I developed signs of another low-level bacterial infection. As a result I was given antibiotics and the Hickman line was immediately removed under local anaesthetic. I had grown to love that Hickman. And once more the infection cleared up.

One afternoon during this second round of chemo I triggered

off another code blue emergency. One of my favourite nurses was injecting antibiotics into my hand. Ouch and more ouch. It really, really hurt, my blood pressure dropped and I again passed out for a few seconds for a rest from the pain. In response to the alert all my medical team raced to my bedside but by this time I was alright. The third time I triggered the code blue I would not be alright.

Sometimes, actually most of the time, boredom set in but it is not right to make the nurses worry. One morning the nurse came in and asked if she could do my obs. I decided to have a bit of mindless pleasure at her expense and said 'no.' I instantly felt regret. Her face fell as she tried to work out how to deal with this once favoured, now recalcitrant patient. I could see her thinking – nurses, we have a problem. She has gone rogue. Of course I declared I was joking. The nurses have a strict routine to follow. Start messing with their minds and the outcome may not be pretty. Although when you get woken up at god knows what hour by someone needing blood from your arm and you don't have a Hickman it is no picnic.

I found out I could play with the oxygenation levels during obs. The aim was for the machine to read 100%. If my level was say 98%, which was still a respectable reading, some quick heavy breathing could bring it up. Job done.

Needles and medical procedures still scared me. I'm not quite sure how, but I learned to deal with it. Repetition and desensitisation I suppose. I had no other choice.

A PICC line (another type of catheter) was now installed in my arm by the radiology team. The visit to radiology was a welcome change of scene. It was an outing. I loved the fresh air after the double-filtered atmosphere of the ward.

Because the hospital routine held no surprises I was much less stressed this time round. I hoped this round of chemo had finally knocked off the dodgy cells. I thought it wouldn't be long before I left for home again.

FOUR

ICU – I see you, but not very well

25 May: Happy days. It looked like I was finally going home after the second round of chemo. But not so fast! I was all dressed up but going nowhere. My temperature had registered 38°C the previous night. I could hardly be bothered getting dressed and had little energy. The nurse took my temperature again. I had cracked a fever. It now registered 39°C. A bad number. She knew something was seriously wrong. I'm later reminded of the Thompson Twins lyrics, 'Oh, Doctor, Doctor, can't you see I'm burning'.

The last thing I remembered was asking the nurses to please, please make me unconscious. I've had enough. I can't stand it anymore. My wish was granted.

Forget about looking forward once more to lying around at home. My body had gone crazy fighting off a serious blood infection. It was fighting itself rather than the invaders.

Sepsis and the Intensive Care Unit here I come.* My life now hung by a thread. I was put into an induced coma and would not be recalling anything that happened during the next week. I was incredibly fortunate to be in the ward when the sepsis hit and not away from the hospital.

Fred takes up the narrative:

I arrive at 7 East and look into the room. I can't yet see Cathy – she is surrounded by at least six doctors and nurses. The PICC line is being taken out, very quickly. This does not look good. The staff part for a moment and my eyes meet Cathy's. She looks frightened and confused. Eventually I enter the room and I am told that she needs to be transferred to a ward where she can be monitored more carefully. ICU is not actually mentioned at this time although that is where she is going. Maybe they don't want to alarm me. I am then told that I need to wait until she is 'settled in' so I decide to go out to Thomastown to collect some didgeridoos for the concert I am working on. About an hour later I am driving back into town and my phone rings. It's The Alfred checking my whereabouts. I am told to come straight up to ICU and meet with some doctors. Now I am pretty nervous about what is going on. I arrive at ICU and two doctors introduce themselves and usher me into a room off the ICU waiting room. They start to explain where thing are at. My heart is pounding as I start to get very worried as to what's coming. They tell me Cathy's infection is serious, and with her zero level immune system, she may not survive the night and I need to be prepared for that possibility. I am overwhelmed with emotion and tears stream down my face. I am trying to

---

* Sepsis is a life-threatening emergency with an estimated mortality rate of between 28% and 50%. In patients with severe sepsis every hour of delay in antimicrobial administration is associated with a 7.6% reduction in survival.

process this extraordinary change of direction. Some hours ago Cathy was coming back to the flat, and now she could die overnight. The doctors are gentle and calming. They have done this before. They warn me I might be shocked by all the tubes and machines around her. I enter the ward. It is pretty quiet. I walk past some rooms. All the patients seem asleep or unconscious. I enter Cathy's room. She seems to be asleep, but she is in an induced coma. Monitoring screens, tubes and wires are everywhere. A ventilator takes over her breathing. It's very confronting. I stand there for a moment trying to take it all in. The nurse explains that she is on a drip of antibiotics, but until they establish exactly what the infection is, it's killing everything. A massive amount of noradrenaline is being administered to treat a life-threatening drop in blood pressure. I draw up a chair, sit and hold her hand. How did we get to this?

All my bodily functions had begun to fail. Only a bank of hi-tech machinery, drugs and the skill of the doctors and nurses were keeping me alive. One of the nurses commented to Fred that these machines only do a tiny proportion of what the human body does to keep us alive every day.

Fred wrote to everyone:

Sunday 27 May.

Well it has been a long 24 hours. Cath is still very sick but there have been some positive things happening thru the day. By this evening they had been able to reduce the blood pressure drug by 50% and blood pressure was still maintaining a good level at this amount. Good. (She is still on a high dose though.) Her temperature had reduced to an almost normal level. Good.

Not too good… she is on dialysis now. Whether there is kidney damage is not known – but usually the kidneys recover – here's hoping.

They will probably take out the ventilator and take her off sedation sooner rather than later. Again, there is a lot to weigh up re timing of this. She is on a load of antibiotics and other drugs.

So – she is still getting a lot of medical support – things have not gone backwards today – more a little forwards. It is positive at the moment but the situation is still serious.

The ICU team are amazing. They take my breath away.

All your prayers, wishes, chanting and thoughts are making a difference.

She is a strong and beautiful person. Your love is sustaining her (and me!)

Fred

Family and friends visited, with none sure if it was the last time they would see me. After Mum saw me I'm told she said, with an edge of sadness and resignation, Well, that's that then. As a teenager she lived under five years of the German occupation of her country during the Second World War, and later coped with the sudden death of my father. There was a real possibility I might die. This was Mum's way of accepting that possibility, of saying goodbye, of coming to terms. I'm so sorry she had to go through that.

Our close friend Tim hopped onto the next plane to leave from northern NSW and, along with our friend Damian, took on the role of Fred's supporter, his shadow.

Monday 28 May.

Well today has seen more small steps in the right direction.

Specifically:

1. *The drug to maintain blood pressure [noradrenaline] has now been reduced to 7 (from 60 on Saturday!) and she is maintaining BP [blood pressure] quite well.*

2. *Her temp. is stable.*

3. *They have identified the bug – it is E. coli – and they can now target it specifically.*

4. *There has been an improvement in her liver and kidney function.*

5. *She is still on dialysis.*

6. *They have halved the sedative – and she is more responsive – but still asleep. When I talked about Gus (our cat) to her she moved her body quite suddenly!*

7. *She is unlikely to remember anything from the ICU experience (mercifully).*

8. *They may remove the ventilator soon – and stop sedatives.*

So – doctors are quite happy. She is stable – with no fluctuations – which is good. They actually used the word excellent when talking and reviewing this evening. She is still in a serious condition – but way better than Saturday (the word relative springs to mind). Next few days will hopefully see this continuing – a long road ahead but moving slowly in the right direction.

Fred

Tuesday 29 May.

Today saw a general slow continuation in the forward direction. Doctors decided it was time to take off the sedation at around 1.00pm. They want to wake her up to a degree at least, although will not be taking out the breathing tubes. At 10.30pm tonight she was still asleep, although I have been told that the drug she has been taking is a long lasting one, and can take 12 hours or more to be filtered away.

As the evening wore on her breathing rate increased dramatically and they decided to put her on another drug that would slow this down. A result of growing consciousness and awareness. It is all a fine dance of drugs, support and interventions – and a lot of waiting. They will wake her up tomorrow, and I imagine as she regains awareness of the tubes down her throat this will not be nice. Most patients find it pretty intolerable needless to say. They can sedate her again quickly though if she stresses too much.

She remains on dialysis – and will for a time yet. Her kidney and liver function have improved slightly again, and they will soon want to see how her kidneys function on their own accord. At present they are not doing much as the machine has taken all this over.

So another day of small gains – it all seems so painfully slow. She continues to be stable – and over the coming 24 hours they will reduce some of the support to gauge how she copes. The staff are amazing – extraordinary skills and care. Have had endless lessons and discussions about treatments, drugs etc. etc. We wait to see what tomorrow will bring – it is still a long way to go. I suspect she will be in ICU for at least another week, maybe longer, before going back to a normal ward.

Fred

At this stage I was still unconscious. Fred continued to describe the situation.

Wednesday 30 May.

Hi All,

Today and this evening thing have continued their slow progression.

Tonight Cathy was beginning to slowly start to wake up. I expect by tomorrow she will be partially conscious for the staff to do some assessments. That will hopefully lead to the removal of the tubes down her throat soon. They have been progressively lowering the amount of support over the past 24 hours, and things have remained pretty stable.

The plan is to have her breathing unassisted soon. The noradrenaline is now at its lowest so far and she seems to be maintaining reasonable pressure. They will be doing some scans tomorrow to do some investigation around where this E. coli bug has possibly come from. Really about eliminating possibilities. Dialysis continues... Liver was under a lot of stress when all this broke loose – hopefully that is not compromised – should be OK though.

It feels like being in a time warp on some strange space ship floating in some universe somewhere!

So – that's about the gist for now.

Fred

It was finally time for this sleeping beauty to wake up. It was not my fate to die in a coma with a multitude of tubes and lines protruding from my body like a high-tech octopus at the age of fifty-nine.

Saturday 2 June.

Sorry for the delay in emails – a lot going on.

Well there have been some big moves.

Friday night she did start to really wake up – and answered in the affirmative by nodding to my question, 'Are you my girl?'

From Sat morning it was clear she was coming up into consciousness. She was opening her eyes and responding to questions from doctors and me. She was clearly desperate to get the breathing tubes out – and they said this could probably happen in the afternoon.

In fact, this happened around 1.00pm – and made a huge difference. She could finally communicate – despite her voice hardly being there at the moment – she can whisper slowly with effort. She is very, very fragile and weak. Later in the arvo the dialysis machine was turned off and we now all hope that her kidneys kick in. This will be monitored overnight. Her other vitals are all pretty good.

She has a feeding tube inserted into her stomach via her nose.

She has made some comments about weird colours and memories – no doubt she will be able to talk more about this as the days go on. She has been desperately thirsty, but can only have liquids via large cotton swabs to ensure she does not aspirate the liquids. She wants out badly but I think she will be in ICU for a few days yet. Last night she was generally calm but started to become anxious late in the evening – and was able to have some mild sedative to take the edge of this.

So – today Saturday – hopefully things will continue to improve. I do feel that she is unable to have any visitors at this time – and will keep you all in the loop with her progress via these emails. Hopefully once she is back in 7 East, some visits can start. As I have said, she is terribly fragile and weak at the moment. She has lost a lot of weight over the week, and her face is gaunt. I was a little shocked once all the tubes and mask etc. had been removed as to how much she has lost – but I am sure this will change over the coming weeks as she begins to eat again.

Fred

The weird world of ICU

As I came out of the induced coma (which took a long two days after the drugs were stopped), and for a day or two afterwards, I had the weirdest ideas, thoughts and delusions which I can still call to mind quite vividly. At first I was inside a beautiful, surreal, huge art work. Incredible Salvador Dali-esque patterns and swirls in orange and bright blue were inside my bedazzled brain. Nothing made any sense. Nothing came together. Where was I? Was it a fever dream? The conscious level of my brain failed to work. (In his book, *Patient: The True Story of a Rare Illness*, English musician Ben Watt described a similar hallucinatory experience. On emerging from a drug-induced sleep for four days in ICU he imagined he was circling above the room, then, along with his partner and mother, he had become part of a painting.) I heard somebody shouting at me. 'Wake up! Wake up!' Maybe I will, maybe I won't. I was too out of it to respond and didn't care anyway. Time to go back inside my artwork.

As I became more conscious of my surroundings the ICU became incorporated into my fantasy world. The feelings all centred on a struggle to get to a place of normality. At the time comedian Dawn French was featuring in a supermarket ad on TV. In my mind she became my nurse, my best mate, my smiling protector, deftly administering finger prick blood tests which I happily succumbed to. Over and over again. My high-tech room turned into a weird, dreamlike railway carriage. I was travelling like mad in the countryside but I couldn't reach the end of the line. I found myself in my hospital bed next to a mob of brown cattle on the open deck of a freighter which was travelling about; going nowhere in a murky world of half-darkness. Then I was travelling in a post-WWII hospital train carriage with hospital beds with high sides lined up in rows. My bed had the words Alfred Hospital in gorgeous, ornate Art Nouveau plastic lettering hanging off the railing. I heard people discussing the Second World War and how to deal with me. I did not fit into their plans.

Then I was trapped by a drug affected art dealer in a massive room with walls thirty feet high. All the walls were covered in magnificent artworks. The dealer floated through the air and offered to sell me this art. I told him they were too big for me to take home. He then tried to kill me. I managed to get away though the powers of my mind.

Some of the dreams mirrored the hospital situation. I had to save my family from being attached to a beeping medical contraption resembling a dialysis machine which would hurt, if not kill, those who get near it. It was as big as a refrigerator but I tried to move it anyway.

In the ICU a clever, and expensive, high tech system turned the clear glass wall to the next room opaque at the touch of a button. It evolved in my mind into a screen slamming shut in my head, preventing me from getting near the elixir which would make me normal again.

Passing through the railway carriages one day I came across an African nurse in colourful traditional clothing which included a patterned scarf wrapped neatly around her head. She was grinding corn in a pestle and mortar and she would not share any corn with me. In reality the nurse was compounding my medicines in a pestle and mortar and putting them down a tube. I could feel the potion running down my nose and throat. In another delusion a patient was bouncing a ball over and over again outside the train carriage. The rhythmic sound of the dialysis machine pumping away had penetrated right into my brain.

But slowly I made more sense of my surroundings.

Fred asked me how long I thought I'd been under. I had no idea but thought I had better be a good girl and give him an answer so guessed seven hours. I saw him go quiet. The next day he told me it was seven days. At least I had the seven correct. I learnt that machines had taken over all my vital functions – there were tubes for breathing, food delivery, dialysis, drugs.

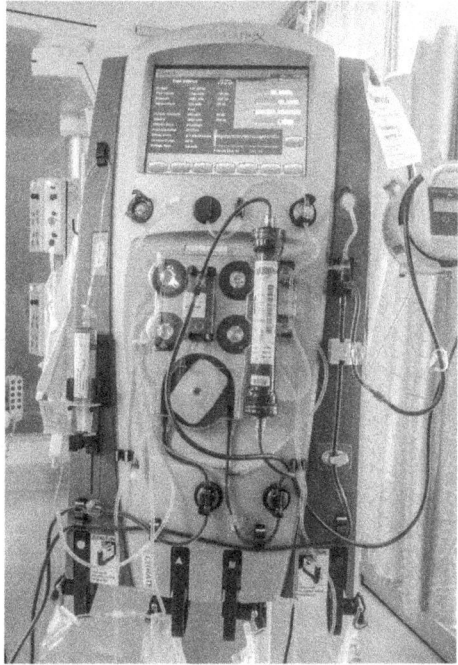

My dialysis machine in ICU

I was so thirsty. Fred told me I was not allowed to drink from a cup as I might choke. He was being silly. I was fine, good to go. I was not going to choke. He gave me a giant earbud dipped in water to suck on. I could hardly lift my head. More please. He gave me a little more. I made a plan in my mind to steal and guzzle an entire glass of water behind Fred's back.

ICU was a surreal place. The night time could be the most challenging time as the atmosphere was even more unreal than during the day. The nurses seemed to walk around like somnambulists. I was sure they must be hypnotised. One night I told the nurse that I was really, really afraid. He chatted with me which helped a little. When I couldn't sleep the nurses gave me a strong sleeping tablet which only worked for four hours, when I found myself wide awake again and feeling frustrated.

Sometimes the tablets did not work at all. I had to ask for another, which could only be obtained with special permission from the doctor. The doctor said yes to another four hours.

Paranoia set in. Another mental miscarriage. I asked Fred the date. Surely it was sometime around my birthday, 27 June. (If you follow astrology my star sign happens to be Cancer. Like the crab I am a skilled homemaker, I have a hard exterior covering up a deeply loving, sensitive nature, like to manoeuvre sideways, change my mind and employment a lot and desire creativity. Cancers are also moody and sensitive, unlike any of the other star signs who are always in a good mood and hard as nails.)

'Saturday 2nd June,' he answered.

'You lie; that cannot be true. No way. Prove it.'

Luckily for him he found the day's newspaper in his bag. Yes, 2 June.

For a second I pondered how I could have been so far ahead of myself date wise. It left me quite puzzled.

Fred told me he gave permission for my participation in a research project comparing filters in the dialysis machine. I didn't trust him to have my best interests at heart and told him so. I didn't spend too much time worrying about it though. My memory was fuzzy and everything he said was only urgent at that moment. My brain was obviously scrambled like Scrabble letters in a velvet bag. Toxins had built up after taking all the drugs and the lack of proper kidney function.

I'm ashamed to say I abused a lovely nurse from South Africa. 'You are crazy to be doing this sort of work,' I said. 'All you do is torture people. Why don't you quit, get a better job and let me get out of here. Just leave me alone or else help me to leave. Please, please, I need to get out. Help me escape.' OK, my request was ludicrous. I did not even know where my clothes were and was lucky to know my name. My addled brain was doing the talking and thank goodness she knew this. She had heard it all before.

The routine continued. There were daily chest X-rays to

check for phlegm collecting in my lungs; a real issue when you are bedridden. Potential chest infections such as pneumonia could kill me. ICU was also a noisy place. The non-stop beeping of all the equipment keeping me alive drilled into my brain. The lights were always on but thankfully they were turned down at night. Just like on the ward, I grabbed sleep when I could. Each morning the doctors, led by a consultant (not the Professor but ICU specialists), did the rounds. They came across as business-like and serious. Questions came my way and the worry was, if I sound like an idiot, I thought they might keep me there longer for non-compliance. On one of the visits the specialist said I did not look well in what sounded to Fred like an accusing voice. The interns looked a bit stunned. I thought about answering, Well, what do you expect? This is ICU and I'm half dead, but I held back. Mum once told her doctor he had a poor bedside manner. Wish I could have seen the look on his face when she said that.

On one occasion I alerted the nurse to the fact that one of my cannulas had fallen out. She didn't seem too worried from my spaced out perspective. Another time, when Fred was visiting, one of the doctors decided to take a cannula out of my arm himself. I must have been drugged up to the eyeballs because I did not care; no needle phobia here. One thing I learned in hospital is that there is a serious art to cannula insertion and removal, with some of the nurses being the go to people for these procedures. As he removed it blood spurted up into a huge gusher and pooled all over the floor. To his embarrassment, and the amusement of the nurses, he had to ask for assistance. 'I won't hear the end of this for days,' he commented.

My appetite was still diminished and as Fred commented I became quite thin; the only food which appealed was small plastic containers of custard. I still had a tube in my nose for feeding. It looked like a taped up rhinoceros horn. Well, it was my job to keep the rhino theme going no matter what. For some reason a lovely memory was triggered. When I ran my gardening business one of my staff stuck a rose thorn on her nose and it too looked like a rhino horn; we all enjoyed a big laugh with her that day. The ICU dietician promised my horn/tube could come out if I ate well. She ordered energy boosting protein drinks. I took a few sips and then lost interest.

I was taken on an outing. Not to the zoo or the park, but to the sunny window looking out at the impressive air ambulance helicopter landing pad. And no, not on foot but wheeled there in my bed. To me any outing was special. We passed the burns ward. Fred looked into the rooms of unfortunate patients who are lying there badly injured and bandaged up. I could not see them easily from my bed.

One aspect of intensive care which can feel undignified is toileting. Occasionally, after a great deal of struggle, I was able to manoeuvre myself to use a bowl. Generally the accepted procedure was to go in your bed. This was one aspect I did not stress about. I had just had a near death experience and couldn't make it to the bathroom if I tried. I was too weak to sit up properly let alone walk. The bedsheets with a protective absorbent pad under the sheets had become my giant nappy. I was attended to promptly by being systematically 'turned' and given fresh sheets. The used sheets were gathered up by male staff members who looked away while a female nurse gave me a thorough wash, even drying the inside of my ears. I felt so good afterwards. It was sheer pleasure. Once I was all cleaned up and the bed expertly remade I was repositioned and propped up with pillows to avoid bedsores. However, I would always slide back into my favourite position – flat on my back. And yes, over the weeks I did get two small sores.

With urination a catheter was inserted painlessly into my bladder and the urine went straight into big see-through plastic bag. I had no sensation at all of needing to pee. The colour, the amount (and the composition?) were checked regularly. It came out a dark yellow colour which indicated my kidneys still had some work to do to get back to normal.

ICU did have its pleasures and plenty of time to take it all in. I found enjoyment in the details of the recently-constructed space-age design; looking at the many uneaten food containers which were lining up on the Corian benchtop; the elegant way the light blue 'privacy' curtains had been designed with scribbly swirls; glancing up at the huge light well as the night closed in above me and looking through those weird glass windows between rooms which became opaque at the touch of a switch.

Massages

Another pleasure was massage. Fred and Damian regularly massaged my legs (I called it rubbing me up the long way). Everybody should experience this. If visitors to your sickbed ask what they can do for you and you know them well enough, suggest either a half-hour foot – or neck rub. It is a real lifesaver and I could not get enough. To avoid blood clots special socks were put on me; it reminded me of my calves being compressed by those heavy black massage chairs at Southern Cross Station. At times I grew sick of the tight socks pumping away, took them off and did not tell the nurses. It was usually ages before they found out and put them back on again.

On the back foot

Fred reported some progress from ICU Central (after three weeks).

17 June.

Well things are moving along – always slowly but ever moving. It looks like she will be back in the ward in the next day or two. We are just waiting for a bed to become available.

...she gains a little more strength each day and today she

was up sitting in a chair for quite some time. It will be a week or two before she can walk easily, but she has made great progress over this past week.

Her kidneys remain a problem – and she will now continue to have dialysis three times a week for 4 hours a time. Hopefully they will repair over coming weeks – we can only hope!

Her spirit is strong – but it does get a battering from time to time – but her humour is there, and I feel certain that over the coming weeks she will continue to gain strength.

I will let you know when she is up to some visits – may be another week yet though.

Your messages and support continue to support and sustain her.

With thanks, Fred

The waiting game continued. As I lay there it struck me as bizarre that I had gone through all this drama in ICU but it had no effect on the leukaemia cells. They were still running amok in my body. First the blood cancer and then the blood infection. Why did I have all these problems with my blood?

19 June.

Well yesterday things seemed to go a little pear-shaped – but I hasten to add that today all seems OK. Won't go into too much detail but there was a worrying bleeding development that was very distressing. After visits from gastro specialists and other doctors, they surmised it was the result of long-term neutropenic-ness (no such word I imagine). They will do some further investigation in a week or two to look for its source.

The best news is that she is going back to Ward 7 East today

– after 24 days in ICU. We are almost back to where she was three weeks ago. Anyway, Cathy is very, very pleased as it is a big boost for her confidence. She is not able to walk yet – hopefully over this week we can attack this. She will be having dialysis in the renal ward three times a week (for 4 hours) for the time being.

So finally we move on again.

Best.

Fred

Farewell ICU

The gastro incident Fred mentioned was confronting. A strange fluid poured out of my body like there was no tomorrow, like I was turning inside out. Surprising really as I had hardly eaten a thing.

It was now home to seventh heaven, base camp, Ward 7 East.

Weird and unusual events can happen when you least expect them. That night of 19 June, the first night back in the ward, was memorable. Around 9 pm an earthquake hit. Yes, the magnitude 5.4 earthquake which had struck in East Gippsland was felt in Melbourne; apparently this earthquake was the strongest recorded in Victoria in three decades. Lying in bed on the seventh floor, I became aware of the building moving in a churning motion. Everything became unstable for some seconds. I had experienced earth tremors in Tokyo (the lights were swinging in the office building across from our hotel but no-one inside took any notice) so had an idea of what was happening. The nurses took time to respond to my buzzer. I suppose they were more than a little surprised themselves and were busy with all the other patients asking them what the hell was happening. Was this a sign of what I had been through?

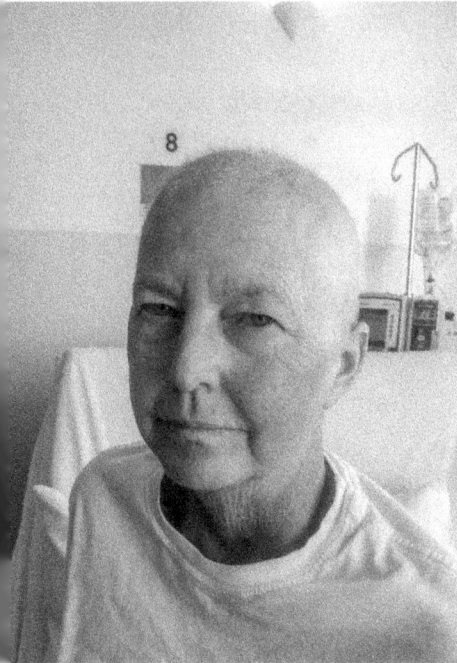

Defiant on 20 June.

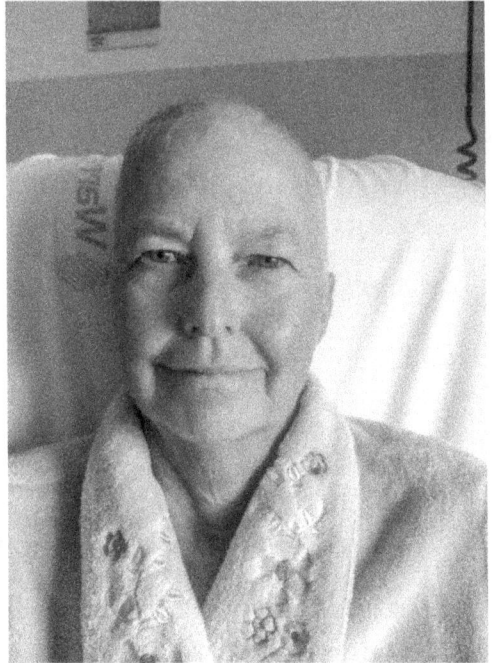

Looking happier the next day.

The world had moved that was for sure. The next day I spoke to Mum on the phone, if you could call it speaking. My voice was still raspy. It was good to talk with her. She told me she had recently undertaken a test for Alzheimer's. I asked her what her score was. 'One out of ten,' I suggested? Sorry Mum, didn't know where that crack came from. Luckily she did not hear me. She was too busy chatting away. For the record, she scored ten out of ten.

Fred took a photo of me which offered a surprise. I looked nowhere near as sickly as I expected. My hair had grown into a grey stubble and my skin looked somewhat off-colour but my cheeks were rosy. I gazed into the camera with a strong, resilient, defiant stare.

The reality was I was angry and totally over it. I could not take any more procedures. The nurses tried three times to do a blood test but my veins had gone on strike. I was perversely proud they have gone into hiding and were not coming out to be stabbed any time soon. I was starting to flip out. Fred became my champion, my advocate. He let the staff know I urgently needed a Hickman or PICC line. The doctor said no. There were patients with more urgent needs than mine. That seemed fair enough but weirdly, on receiving this news I was totally calm because I was certain, without any proof, there would be a cancellation. Sure enough, the next morning I was told someone had cancelled and I could get a PICC. I hoped the bloody thing wouldn't get blocked.

Food wise, Fred and the nurses encouraged me to eat and I tried my best to please them. My desire for food continued to be low. The energy drinks still kept appearing with each meal and I accumulated a nice stack of them on my bedside table, almost enough to start a milk bar. But I was not drinking them. Well, just a few sips to please my team.

Re-learning how to walk

An even bigger issue now reared its head – I still couldn't walk. Fred's words rang in my ears and became implanted there. I can help you with a lot of things to make your situation a bit better but I can't walk for you. I'm sorry, *only you* can learn to walk again. Two friendly physiotherapists came to get me out of bed. No, I could not do it. It is a strange sensation to describe if you haven't experienced it yourself. My entire body felt out of sync, discombobulated. My centre of balance had shifted to the wrong place. Maybe it had moved out of my body entirely. I felt so envious of every person I saw who was capable of walking – the cleaners, the staff delivering afternoon tea, the doctors, the physiotherapy staff, Fred. How come they could walk and I couldn't? I was jealous of everyone in the entire world who was mobile. I managed to walk a few steps, gingerly putting one foot in front of the other. I made it to the door and straight back to my bed.

Next task – sitting for a long time in a chair. It was hard to hold myself up; horizontal was my new normal. Sitting in a chair used to be a totally automatic activity. Not on this day. I stood up in a wobbly way. I tried to balance on one leg but could only do it for a few seconds. My bed had become my sanctuary. I couldn't wait to get back into its warm embrace.

FIVE

Life after ICU
– Rehabilitation

Rehab is not only for alcoholics and drug addicts. It is also for people like me who can't walk because they have undergone two rounds of chemo followed by more than three weeks flat on their backs in ICU. The best thing about being transferred to Caulfield Hospital was that the ward had marvellous fresh air. The other patients in my room were both men and women; patients came and went and most were not interested in small talk. Some didn't speak at all. One woman I did talk to had seriously hurt herself when crashing onto the bitumen road during a bike race.

Going to the hospital gym was like being inside a Fellini movie. We were all damaged in some way and making the best of it. There were patients of various ages and sizes, some large, some thin. Some were missing a limb or two, recovering from bad accidents or had a brain injury. The attendant delivered me there and back by wheelchair. Walking along the low parallel bars and getting to the end was a huge achievement, as was walking up a few steps and back down again and lying down doing stretching exercises. For the first time ever, I used a rowing machine and enjoyed it.

A small victory was being well enough to receive visitors. Just getting from my room to the lounge/eating area to spend time with them was a challenge. My energy levels were still low and only built up in small increments each day. The hospital had extensive grounds. Fred took me for a spin in the wheelchair via the coffee shop. Somehow, I managed to walk almost all the way around the complex. Quite an improvement on the five steps I took to the door of my room at The Alfred not long before.

Colonoscopy

Because of intestinal bleeding during the second round of chemo, the doctor ordered a colonoscopy. The worst thing about this procedure was the drink spiked with a substance which totally cleaned the bowel out. It tasted unappealing; you have to take glasses and glasses of the stuff and the ultimate result – ten trips to the toilet. A more enjoyable trip was back to The Alfred by ambulance; quite a novel experience. No sirens blazing though.

I can recommend the twilight-type sedative administered for the colonoscopy. I think it is called Propofol. It had a similar effect to the drug given for bone marrow biopsies and for all I know may be the same drug. I did not recollect the actual procedure and afterwards felt elated. I didn't have a care in the world. Global warming? Your point is? Plastic pollution in the oceans? That's alright but I'm hungry, please get me a cheese sandwich. If you can grill it for me all the better. The cancer cells still hiding out and multiplying away in my body? We will talk about that later.

That euphoric feeling did not last of course. A wave of paranoia hit me after Fred left. I was taken to another ward, rather than back to Caulfield, in order for some blood levels to be checked. It was now night-time and I was in a room by myself. Oh no, it was horrifying. I thought I must have been adult-napped. My treatment regime seemed to be going into reverse. I was back in hospital and the doctors were going to keep me here! Quick, push the buzzer. By this time I was in tears. 'Nurse, please help me. I'm so frightened.' She reassured me the stay was only for the night and I would be returned safe and sound to Caulfield the next day. What a relief. Dodged a bullet there. I felt so delicate and fragile.

Home again

After more days of rehab I was fit enough to go back home to the flat at Xavier College. I followed up with a few sessions at the Royal Talbot Rehabilitation Centre in Kew. My status at The Alfred again changed from inpatient (or maybe I should say impatient) to outpatient. I visited often for a check of my blood levels followed by a top up of blood, magnesium or plasma (or for another bone marrow biopsy). Thank you blood donors. With my needle issues the last thing I could do in the past was give blood. I asked Professor Curtis if the Blood Bank would take my blood if I was cured, but no, it was not up to standard. My blood was not worth bottling. I am on the organ donor register and planned to donate my organs after death if the circumstances were right. They are probably not much use now either.

Plan B

As it turns out, the two rounds of chemotherapy had not cured the AML. Some microscopic residual cells showed up on the next bone marrow biopsy, still acting like it was party time. They were running about the place with plans to multiply and finish off their unwilling host. This started me thinking. Do cells have intelligence? Can they really party and plan? They certainly can run amok and turn into killers when your back is turned, that I do know.

So, the options were stark.

Option 1:   Do nothing and probably die within a few days, weeks or months.

Option 2:   Have more chemotherapy and possibly die from the side effects.

Option 3:   Have a stem cell transplant and possibly die from complications, or be fortunate enough for it to work.

The cut off age for a transplant is not set in stone.

The thought of more hospital procedures did not excite me. Apart from those feral white blood cells my general health was good. Professor Curtis offered me option three as a possibility and I chose it.

Time for me to send an email for once:

Thought I'd give Fred a break and send everyone a medical update myself, now that I am regaining my energy and coming to terms with the small c journey which started with the 29 March diagnosis. Apologies to those who have visited, phoned or emailed and have heard the following already!

It's so great to be back at home with Fred (who has been my lifesaver in every way) and seeing family and friends but I'm still working my way back to normality. It will take a while.

It is funny but my diary is pretty full with follow up medical obligations. My red blood production isn't yet back to normal so I received a blood transfusion yesterday. My PICC port is dressed in outpatients weekly and I'm attending weekly rehab at Royal Talbot and seeing a chiropractor. I've also seen the Professor regularly as he is overseeing my stem cell transplant which I have decided to go ahead with. I figure since the transplant is on offer and should increase my chances of survival into the future, I should proceed.

The transplant will be happening mid-September... Prior to the procedure, I have to undergo quite a few tests... the PICC line taken out and a Hickman line put in. The taking of marrow from the donor is a bit more uncomfortable than putting it into me as it goes straight into my Hickman port. The donor has to have a series of injections to stimulate the marrow before it is taken out a bit like a blood transfusion. I will have a mild dose of chemo tablets to supress rather than eliminate my immune system and will have radiation on the transplant day. My [anonymous] donor is from Australia. Then its lots of drugs to suppress immunity so that the marrow can take over and kill off any cancer cells. Hopefully there won't be any complications, which can happen.

I asked the Professor about my chances of survival. How many times has he had to answer that question? About a million times I imagine. He replied '100% either way. You have a 100% chance of living and a 100% chance of dying.' That made me smile. According to the Leukaemia Foundation, in Australia, the five-year survival rate for AML is 27% for adults. [The five-year survival rate for children is around 70%.] It doesn't say if this is with or without a stem cell transplant.

I was interested to find that I will take on the donor's blood type, will be making enough red blood cells and will lose immunity to childhood diseases. The process will take place as an outpatient. I've spoken to someone who had it done and she was happy with the transplant although awfully tired for the first two months.

As you can see I'm totally preoccupied with the world of medicine!

I hope you are all well and happy.

Love Cathy

SIX

The stem cell transplant

The decision to have a stem cell transplant was not to be taken lightly. I thank my lucky stars for our medical system, where the offer of a transplant did not mean having to sell our house or declare bankruptcy. Professor Curtis made some salient points about stem cells in an online interview:

The interesting aspect of stem cells is that they can divide and generate mature cells and generate cells which are identical to itself. That cell or its progeny or daughters or brothers can be maintained for the life of that person. That's why bone marrow transplants work; we collect the stem cells from one patient and give it to another person who has leukaemia. The stem cells allow the new blood cells to grow and keep growing – the property of self-renewal. These cells can differentiate, make white and red blood cells to carry oxygen. But they can't turn into any other cell types.

* Professor David Curtis. Up Close interview, University of Melbourne, Episode 93: What Role Stem Cells in Leukaemia?

There was a one in four chance of siblings having the same tissue type which makes for the best genetic match. My brothers, Peter and John, were tested but both were a mismatch. However, from the test John discovered he had type 2 diabetes, (it runs in my family), which he could now take steps to control.

The next procedure for me was an allogenic stem cell transplant. The anonymous donor is the real hero of this story. Healthy stem cells are donated from another unrelated person, a genetically matched donor, to replace the patient's unhealthy ones. The white blood cells of the donor's immune system are collected and transplanted along with their stem cells. It is hoped these cells will attack and destroy all traces of the underlying disease. A search was made in the registries in Australia and overseas to find my genetic twin. As a Caucasian I had a good chance of a match as 77% of the donors world-wide are white. At present those of African, Asian or Hispanic ancestry or mixed race have far fewer options available to them. Only 3% of donors world-wide are of mixed race which means finding a match is a bit like winning the lottery.

An interesting fact: in 2017-18 The Alfred did twenty-nine allogenic transplants and fifty-six autologous (own cell) transplants.

I had two matches, one in Germany and one in Australia. Ten million potential bone marrow donors are registered in Germany but only 200,000 Australian donors are on the Australian Bone Marrow Donor Registry.

Nurses from The Alfred Hospital regularly travel overseas and interstate to collect the precious donor cells which they keep with them on the plane. (No; the cells do not have their own seat.) The doctors decided to use the stem cells from the Australian donor, a woman aged forty.

Pre-transplant planning and treatment

In the week leading up to the transplant, because of my age and ultimately poor response to the earlier chemo, I received reduced-intensity-conditioning therapy in the form of chemo tablets and radiation to suppress my immune system so that it would accept the donor stem cells.

Here is the impressive list of the procedures undertaken prior to transplant:

· dental X-ray and visit to the dentist

· urine collection and blood test

· bone marrow biopsy with four blood tests including chimerism bloods

· chest X-ray

· ECG

· lung function test

· information session with Nurse Georgia

· Hickman catheter insertion and dressing

· radiation oncologist information and measurement session

· clinical psychologist session

· bone mineral density test

· meeting with the pharmacist followed by four days rest at home taking chemo tablets.

I was also given a detailed brochure to assist in understanding the transplant process and help to adjust to recovery and the new post-transplant world.

My blood counts would drop dramatically in the week following the conditioning therapy.

In addition, I took a stack of tablets for quite some time and hoped the whole experience didn't make me too sick. Immunosuppressants were given to me before, during and for after the transplant to reduce the risk of the donor's stem cells being rejected by my body, along with antibiotics and other drugs prescribed to help prevent or treat infections.

My medication commencing 14 September 2012:

- Fludarabine tablets, an immunosuppressant used for three days prior to transplant

- Cyclosporin capsules to supress the immune system. (Later on this was changed to Tacrolimus, an antibiotic derived from a fungus found in the soil. The warning on the packet advises not to drink too much grapefruit juice, avoid excessive skin exposure to sunlight or drive heavy machinery while on this drug)

- Mycophenolate mofetil tablets to supress the immune system

- Sulfamethoxazole-Trimethoprim tablets to treat bacterial infection

- Valaciclovir tablets to treat or prevent viral infections such as shingles

- Ondansetron tablets for relief of nausea or vomiting

- Peter MacCallum Mouthwash to help mouth ulcers heal

- Metoclopramide tablets as back up for nausea

- Ciprofloxacin tablets antibiotic to treat or prevent bacterial infections, starting when neutrophil levels are less than 0.5.

As I mentioned, the extraction of the stem cells is more uncomfortable for the donor than it is for the patient receiving them. The donor first has to undergo a series of injections to stimulate the peripheral blood stem cells to enter the blood stream. Once they are at a certain level, the donor is attached to a blood cell separator (apheresis machine) where the cells are withdrawn from their blood. One benefit for the donor is a full health check to ensure diseases are not passed on to the patient.

On 21st September, the big day, I had a total body irradiation and another blood test. The donated stem cells were infused through a vein into my blood stream. From here the stem cells made their way to my bone marrow where they became established and commenced making new blood cells. These cells are clever navigators. I wanted to know how they could figure out where my bone marrow was located.

Post-transplant monitoring

Close monitoring pre-and post-transplant was vital. In the first six to twelve months following a transplant survival can be touch and go. Even with all the available science at hand, no-one can confidently predict if the donor cells will make themselves at home. Also, after the chemotherapy and irradiation there is greater risk of infection because of a lack of infection-fighting white blood cells. Between 24 September and 16 October I visited the Haematology Oncology Clinic for ten routine blood tests and a review by the transplant Registrar who orders platelet transfusions as needed and red blood cell transfusions when haemoglobin levels were too low. I saw Professor Curtis four times so he could check my blood counts, see how I was progressing, and deal with any problems that might arise.

Graft versus host disease (GVHD)

Why this intense follow-up? Apart from the chemo's effect on the blood, a common and sometimes life-threatening complication of allogenic (donated) transplants is called graft versus host disease (GVHD), an immune reaction whereby cells from the donor's immune system recognise the patient's body as foreign and attack it. It can lead to organ damage and skin disfigurement. When it develops soon after the transplant, drugs such as steroids are given to further suppress the new immune system and reduce symptoms. However, a small amount of acute GVHD is considered a positive development as the donor's T-cells see any residual cancer cells as foreign and attack them. As I was to discover, GVHD can also develop at a later stage, or persist for months and sometimes years after the transplant. There is a 40% to 80% chance of GVHD symptoms developing (depending on what sources you use).

A new waiting game had begun. I spent lots of time in bed. I was over it and couldn't wait to have new energy. I hoped this transplant worked and didn't want to contemplate the future if it failed.

Slowly but surely, my blood counts started to rise. The new cells were making themselves at home and starting to 'engraft' and hopefully attack any leftover leukaemia cells. I looked forward to what is termed chimerism, a state where 100% of the bone marrow and blood cells in my body was of donor origin, a successful takeover bid. I used to be B positive and now took on the donor's blood type, coincidentally also B positive.

And consider this. Now I am a genetic chimera. The donor's DNA is inside me along with her stem cells. The white blood cells the stem cells produce also have her DNA (red blood cells do not contain DNA because they lack a nucleus). This means a genealogical profile done by organisations such as Ancestry will probably not work. They test DNA collected from a customer's saliva which can include a combination of my own DNA and the DNA of the stem cell donor. If I commit a serious crime, the donor's blood DNA profile might end up on the police data base instead of my DNA. Hmmm. The mind boggles at the idea.

SEVEN

What else can go wrong?

I'm cured!???

There comes a time after the stem cell transplant where, if all goes well, the word cure replaces the word remission. I did not record or pinpoint the first time Professor Curtis told me I was cured of AML. From memory this happened around two years after diagnosis. Although I was glad to hear the word this was not a cure moment. My blood levels were tracking efficiently towards normal so it was more of a progression, not a big surprise. And, cure does not mean the elimination of ongoing side effects of treatment.

The chances of the AML returning were slim but there were challenges ahead.

Vaccinations – back to the beginning

It can take a year or even longer for the immune system to fully recover following the transplant. Because of the risk of infection, precautions have to be taken during this time such as avoiding contact with people with a malady like flu, measles or chicken pox. Because the transplant meant I lost my immunity to all the diseases I was immunised against as a child a series of vaccinations were given against diseases such as polio, tetanus, meningococcus and diphtheria, along with the annual influenza vaccine.

I was struck by an intriguing thought regarding vaccinations. Dad's father and two of his siblings died of tuberculosis in The Netherlands in the 1930s. As a result, the family of seven lost their house and farm and were thrown into poverty. Dad had to leave school and support the family at a young age. How different his teenage years would have been if his family had been vaccinated against TB. He may have been a prosperous farmer in The Netherlands; he would not have migrated and fathered children in Australia. I would have undergone cancer treatment under the Dutch medical system or maybe not had cancer at all.

By the end of 2012 Fred had given up the Xavier College boarding assistant position so we rented out our little country house for a year and moved out of the flat. Early in the new year we settled into Rowland Street, Kew, a beautiful tree-lined street lined with many multi-million dollar houses. Former Prime Minister Gough Whitlam's childhood home, regrettably now demolished, was in this street. Our spacious Californian bungalow had a petite front and back garden. Fruit bats stopped over in one of the trees, and although the birdlife was sparse in comparison to our country place, the odd magpie and crow explored the lawn and garden beds.

Apart from increased likelihood of infection there were other not-insubstantial risks connected to chemo/radiotherapy and the stem cell transplant. These included cardiovascular and lung issues and osteoporosis. The future would become all about continuing to manage the side effects of chronic GVHD and the effects of the drugs I needed to take to control it.

One year after diagnosis – Welcome to Herpes World

In 2013, while working at the computer, I started to feel itchy and tingly down the right side of my back. Was it fleas from the cat or some little bugs in the furniture which had migrated onto my clothing? Another trip to the Outpatient Clinic was required to find out what was wrong. I described the symptoms. Apart from the irritating, prickly skin rash around the right-hand side of my back and torso which turned into small blisters, I felt sluggish and unwell. Oh no! Shingles. A biopsy was needed to confirm the doctor's diagnosis. Another person came in, injected local anaesthetic into my upper thigh and excavated a small sample for testing. Outwardly I showed no distress. Sure enough – shingles. Time for some shingles education.

Shingles is a viral infection caused by the varicella-zoster virus which is a species in the *Herpesviridae* family of DNA viruses. This is the same virus that causes the chickenpox I contracted as a child. The virus then lies around relaxing in nerve tissues near the brain and spinal cord. Because my immune system was underpowered, the virus was reactivated as shingles. Shingles does not kill you. It just makes you feel sick. Potions were prescribed, then back to the haven of bed for a few days and full recovery after four weeks.

I was surprised to learn that around 130 herpes viruses are known, eight of which routinely affect humans. These clever viruses are able to establish lifelong infections by evading the immune system in many different ways. One of the tests I undertook when first admitted to hospital was for human cytomegalovirus (CMV), otherwise known as human herpes virus 5 which is transferred via bodily fluids. Around 75% of the Australian population have this virus dormant in their bodies. If you are healthy CMV goes unnoticed. I had no idea about it before I became sick. The hospital kept an eye on CMV because being immunocompromised can lead to a reactivation of the virus with potentially life-threatening results, hence the Valaciclovir tablets I was prescribed.

Tangles with Gus the cat

One night, 18 months after my transplant, Gus was sleeping on the edge of the bed. The light was off. I visited the bathroom and on my return gave him a pat on the front of his head. Big mistake. He woke up in fright, immediately interpreted this as an assault, turned feral and attacked my arm, then pulled back and attacked again, leaving long, potentially infectious, scratches on my arm. Poor thing, I instinctively gave him a huge kick which flung him right off the bed (he survived without incident). All I could do after that was lie there in the dark thinking, What the heck just happened?

Then two and a half years after the stem-cell transplant, we were spending time in our home in the countryside. Winters can get quite cold in the hills so the cosy wood fire in our lounge room burned day and night. On this night the fire burned more than firewood. Luckily it was on the lowest setting and not cranked right up. I was in my flannelette pyjamas, the top of which had sleeves which only covered two thirds of my arm. I stood next to the fire with Gus near my feet. As I took a step towards the kitchen Gus took fright. The result – my feet and his paws became entangled and I lost my balance. Have you ever felt like time has decelerated, slowing down as you started to fall? I experienced this phenomenon big time as I fell towards the fire. A quick decision needed to be made. Use my hand to break my fall, or use the inside of my lower arm? I chose the lower arm. Instantly, many layers of skin melted over a 15cm long patch of skin as I made contact with the hot metal. A small shock set in and it did not hurt at first. As I ran cool water over the burn, Fred arrived home from the city. Just in time to bandage me up. Over the next days a light-yellow substance wept from the wound and quite a few trips were made to the local medical clinic for regular dressing and antiseptic cream.

My one big worry was that my immune system would be too weak to fight off infection. This turned out to be unfounded. The burn healed nicely and today the large white scar is hardly visible at first glance. As with the scratched arm, no infection resulted. Reassuringly, my immune system worked quite well.

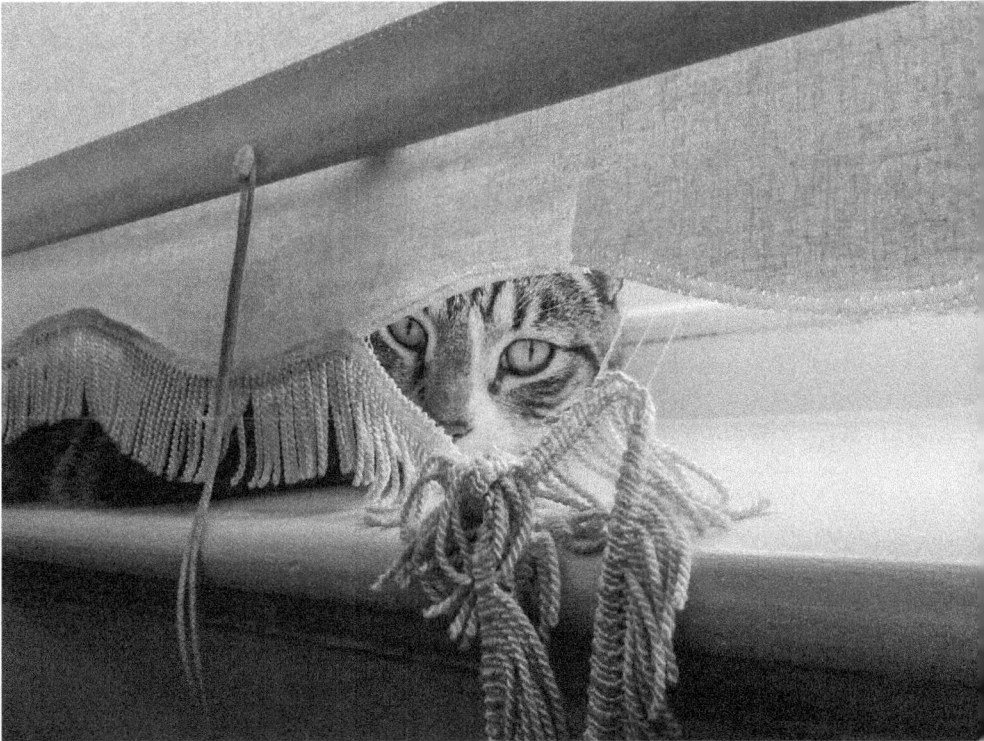

Three years after diagnosis – off the rails with diabetes

Around Christmas 2015, three years after my transplant, I started to feel seriously unwell again. A new kind of sick feeling really kicked in; I was going to the toilet to pee far more than usual and felt terribly thirsty. My skin was dry, my eyes were dull, bad leg cramps plagued me at night and my energy was low all day. Once more walking along the street became a challenge. Fred bought me a voucher for a massage but I felt just as bad afterwards. On top of that my vision had become blurry. I craved lots of sugary foods such as biscuits. My sweet tooth was nothing new. Mum was a skilled baker of pastries; her repertoire varied from lemon meringue pies to Dutch almond cookies and sponges on tap for afternoon tea and homemade ice-cream for dessert. However, this craving had become extreme. I suspected I was turning into a sugar junkie.

GVHD symptoms, especially painful mouth ulcers and lesions, had appeared on and off since the stem cell transplant. It was so annoying to miss out on eating many curries as I could not take the heat of chillies; the inside of my mouth was too sensitive. Another symptom was feeling like I had a cold permanently coming on. A blood test showed the donor cells were again attacking my liver cells as well as mopping up the cancer cells.

Prednisolone, one of the drugs I took to counteract the effects of GVHD, is a powerful type of medicine known as a corticosteroid or steroid which reduces inflammation and damps down the immune system. Although I went around telling people I was 'roided up to amuse myself, my muscle strength was certainly not much chop! I could barely lift a house brick, let alone smash a few up. Prednisolone can have many side effects including fluid retention (no), insomnia (yes), irritability and mood swings (yes), disorientation (yes, sometimes), high blood pressure (no), loss of potassium (no), headache (sometimes), bone density loss as it affects how the body uses calcium and vitamin D to build bones (yes), cataracts (no), weight gain (yes) and swollen face (definitively yes). My face had now swelled up like a puff adder and I couldn't bear to look at myself in the mirror. Prednisolone can also affect the body's response to insulin, bringing on type 2 diabetes and that was what I was now dealing with! Because my pancreas was still working, but not as effectively as it needed to, my body was building insulin resistance and unable to effectively convert glucose into energy leaving too much glucose in the blood. I had earlier experienced some temporary elevation of my blood glucose levels (BGL) after taking Prednisolone.

After Christmas Professor Curtis took one look at my BGL of 28 and put me straight into the ward to get the diabetes and drug levels sorted. In a person without diabetes, BGLs range between 4.0-7.8 millimoles of glucose per litre of blood (mmols/L) throughout the day so a reading of 28 was far too high. I was glad to be back in hospital. However, a big shock came my way. My worst nightmare was about to be unveiled. No, not the cancer coming back, but having to give myself endless finger pricks as well as injections of insulin into my belly. My needle phobia suddenly went to eleven out of ten.

At least my single room in The Alfred Centre with a sitting area and its own bathroom was nice, luxurious in fact. The only problem was, I was too scared to enjoy it, just like I was too sick to truly enjoy my newly svelte, size-ten figure after the chemotherapy.

Specialist teams and individuals visited – the haematology team, the endocrinologists, the pharmacist, the diabetes nurse educator. The social worker took me through Exposure and Habituation therapy, a useful technique devised by therapists at the University of Exeter. It works by putting you in charge of confronting the fearful things you have been avoiding for a lifetime, facing the fear in stages. The hospital routine mirrored the earlier one in 7 East – the food menu to fill in, the cleaner giving the room a tidy up, the occasional volunteer selling newspapers and magazines, the person filling up the water jug.

I had learned an important fact: It was essential to stay hydrated.

The educators and nurses helped me through the routine of blood glucose level testing throughout the day. For those of you fortunate enough not to have diabetes, here is the routine:

It commences with a finger prick with the lancer. I could choose the force with which it goes in, and I naturally chose the setting with the least impact. It still hurt a little bit. The gizmo also told me how many of the six lancers I had already used. (They can be used more than once by the same person but you shouldn't use the same one for months until it goes blunt.)

Put the little globule of bright red blood onto a small strip which has been placed into a hand held meter. A number magically appears. Record the number on a sheet.

Then the big moment – injecting the insulin. There are different kinds of insulin; some are slow release, some fast. Put a new needle onto the tip of the injector device, or pen as the manufacturer calls it. Shake the pen to mix up the insulin. Take off the two safety caps and inject 2mls into the air to check nothing is blocked. Select the correct amount of insulin (I went totally tense at this point). Press the pen against the skin on my belly, break surface skin, inject into the belly and wait six seconds before removing the needle.

This is the step I found incredibly difficult because I was so scared. I held my breath and experienced the fear. I had to do it. The alternative was long-term complications such as loss of vision, kidney or heart disease, or limb amputation. I discovered it did not really hurt at all. Next take the needle from the device using the large safety cap and dispose of it carefully. I repeated the procedure the next day. And the one after that. It was never easy.

It took a few days for the blood glucose level to stabilise. I much preferred to give myself the blood tests and insulin injections rather than receiving them from the nurses. I don't know if they had bigger needles, used more force or if the settings were higher. They seemed to hurt more. Most mornings in the ward I was woken up with a blood test. That certainly made the juices flow for the day. Then it was time to do the blood sugar level test, inject insulin and savour the reward of breakfast. I developed an addiction to vegemite on cheap, fresh white bread. The food had improved since my last stopover, or else my tastebuds had changed. Even the roasts tasted good. Then more BGL testing, insulin, lunch. The insulin was having a beneficial effect. My eyesight was no longer blurry. Another bonus – stronger nails and hair and smooth, hydrated skin. Quite nice, and saved on moisturiser too.

Just when everything settled down one of the doctors gave me a reality check. He told me I could be on insulin for six months. I was shocked. Say it isn't so. In my head I heard Jack Nicholson yelling, 'You can't handle the truth!' The doctor's bland statement of fact felt like the last straw. Why prescribe a drug with such powerful side effects? I had to take drugs to fix the side effects of the drug I was taking to counteract side effects of the transplant. The whole thing struck me as nuts. There was no end in sight. Professor Curtis made me face the facts. GVHD is so much worse than the steroids. GVHD can kill you. I tried my 'roided up phrase on Professor Curtis at my next appointment. He was mildly amused.

The agitation did not subside. After a week's stay at home, I had a massive anxiety attack, a total physical and mental crack up. It was January, the weather was hot and for a time we had a power outage so we couldn't use the air conditioner or even a fan. After a week of giving myself finger pricks and injections my resilience deserted me. All the terrors I experienced during medical procedures as a child and at The Alfred came pouring out. Sleep eluded me. I tossed and turned, quaked and sweated.

I needed to vomit. I stuck my fingers right down my throat but nothing much came up because I could not eat. I became totally dehydrated. No relief. Waves of shaking and quivering washed over me. It was the scariest feeling with no end in sight. I wanted to pass out. The horrible anxiety grew and grew as I became obsessed with thoughts of the next injection. I lay there in fear, sweating in the heat for half an hour before having to administer the insulin. I held my breath, went tense. Then had to inject. No other choice. This time I found little relief in the periods between procedures, no eye in the middle of the cyclone.

Fred was there with me but the only option was to get medical help so I asked him to take me to The Alfred's Emergency Department.

A new terror crept in. Will they think I am being stupid and neurotic and send me back home? Did they have a spare bed given it was still the holidays?

There is a certain irony in the fact I was contemplating voluntarily admitting myself to the place where I was going to be given even more blood tests and needles than at home. If I had not been so anxious in the Emergency Department I would have quietly laughed at my predicament. On arrival the doctor could not find a vein to do a blood test. They probably went into hiding due to dehydration. He was successful after four, yes four, attempts, the last a procedure to insert a cannula so that I could be given fluids. A bit later I noted the fluid was not dripping from the bag down into the tube like it was supposed to. It turned out the drip wasn't working.

A bed was found for me on the cystic fibrosis ward. The hospital routine and the attentions of the doctors and nurses did the trick. The apprehension subsided and injecting insulin became manageable.

You may have noticed I do not have a medical background. However, unless type 2 diabetes is induced by drugs such as Prednisolone or the reading is sky high, I don't think injecting insulin should be the first choice of treatment (type 1 diabetes is a different ball game). Fasting, exercise, weight loss and eating the right foods and even drugs can lower blood sugar levels (and possibly provide a cure?) without stepping on the insulin merry go round.

After a week I was discharged. While in the car on the way home the final few bars of Mahler's *Fifth Symphony* came on the radio. Without warning I wept copious tears and it felt so good. Luckily I was not driving. On the topic of driving a car while diabetic, if you live in the state of Victoria and have (or develop) diabetes you must notify VicRoads, using a form filled in by your doctor, and provide further medical reports if and as requested. And if you don't provide these on time your licence may be suspended. This makes sense safety-wise but I didn't know this was a rule until I developed diabetes myself. My first thought was – more bloody forms to fill in. My second thought was – if I lose my licence there is no way to get to a supermarket if Fred's not here. Our country town only has a small general store with the nearest larger town a twenty-minute drive or an expensive taxi ride away. As it turned out my licence was not affected.

When I returned from hospital Fred had to travel to Adelaide for work. I was not concerned. I had to face the next few days alone and wouldn't be driving anywhere. I spent the first two days experiencing new waves of anxiety every minute or two. I worked out that to let these waves flow over me was the most suitable approach to take. Weirdly, I almost began to enjoy riding the waves rather than resisting the feelings that came up. Relief came, and I was able to function to some extent, in spite of the fact that I could barely sign my name. My hand shook so much my signature looked like a manic spider had trawled across the page. Over the next few weeks the waves slowly subsided. I now injected insulin without totally freaking out. However a vague feeling of general anxiety now enveloped me.

High maintenance

Although withdrawing somewhat from the world, I still made the effort to send an email to a friend in May 2016.

I have gone to ground and have not been very social, quietly dealing with what turned out to be a hard time health-wise…

The last few months I've been slowly weaned off the steroids. The graft versus host has been up and down; there has been quite a fight going on – but finally I have turned the corner. The steroid has been greatly reduced as has the insulin. I'm feeling normal again rather than 60%. And with a new chapter for my leukaemia book (I'm thinking of calling it Cancer Cells or The Leukaemia Cha Cha) – what it is like to get diabetes. Hopefully in the next month or two I will be off the steroids and the plan is for the insulin to stop as well. I have a family history of type 2 diabetes so will have to be careful but the diabetes symptoms should disappear with the drug no longer being taken. The steroids made my face puff up so that wasn't fabulous either.

I carefully recorded my insulin levels for the Diabetes Educators. The haematologist was right. It took six months for the Prednisolone and the insulin dosage to be reduced to zero. At this stage my BGL was now normal. At this stage…

Another house move was made late in 2016, from Kew to a small flat near the city centre, with continued using of our country place as an alternative home. It was easy to visit The Alfred, easy for Fred to commute to Monash University and easy for me to work in a garden. The best of all worlds.

Weird side effects

I noticed some interesting side effects now I had gorgeous new blood. Some perfumes and deodorants, but not all, made me feel nauseous and unwell. Being on an airplane or a tram could feel like being in a chemical soup, with symptoms ranging from sneezing to mild headache and brain fog. This was especially noticeable during our 2016 flight to the States, even though the new Dreamliner we travelled on was promoted as having improved oxygen saturation levels. Being in a cramped nine across seating configuration did not help either. I was excited to breathe LA-style fresh air when we landed.

When I was ill, mosquitoes showed no interest in my second-rate blood and I received far fewer bites than usual. Now that my blood level had returned to normal my attractiveness to mosquitoes ramped up a level. I shared this insight with Professor Curtis, suggesting he could be up for a Nobel Prize for Medicine if he researched this phenomenon further. Surprisingly he expressed doubt as to my theory. I later read there are over 3,000 species of mosquitoes. Most don't bite humans. The myriad of reasons for mosquitoes gravitating to certain people, some more scientifically based than others I must add, include blood type (apparently they prefer Type O), the chemical composition of sweat, drinking beer, the colour of your shirt and the bacteria which lives on skin or proteins in the blood. And maybe the health of your blood?

Late Effects Clinics

Five years after my diagnosis the AML was now well and truly cured. I tried not to worry too much about all the risks and side effects; I dealt with them when they came up. Change in my health status had become par for the course. However, The Alfred does not transplant someone else's cells into you and then say – See you later. Don't call us with your problems.

Potential effects and relevant risk factors are identified at regular Late Effects Clinics. An individualised clinical summary and survivorship care plan is created based on diagnosis, treatments received, side effects as well as medical, family and social history. In other words, a thorough examination of my health status is provided.

Extensive tests and check-ups are undertaken: bloods checked, Pap smear, mammography, bowel screening, thyroid test, heart test, blood pressure, cholesterol, fasting blood glucose, bone density scan, calcium and vitamin D levels, ferritin test for iron level, lung function test, skin cancer check, eye-sight and dental check-ups, vaccinations and last but not least psychosocial wellbeing. A number of these tests are done at clinics or hospitals apart from The Alfred. At my third clinic in 2017 the results were generally excellent, except for osteopenia in the lumbar spine (the stage before osteoporosis), raised cholesterol levels and high iron levels through previous blood transfusions. My blood glucose level improved as the steroids were reduced and were now generally within acceptable range. Surprisingly, I only had two bouts of the common cold in the previous five years.

A symptom of concern was listed – a lesion on left side bridge of nose requiring dermatological assessment. A horrid wart-type growth appeared and it kept growing which made me feel self-conscious. The lovely staff at the skin cancer clinic gathered together and consulted. A biopsy was required, involving a local anaesthetic. By now I had become even more desensitised to needles. I had no further energy to expend on worrying about it and could have blood tests and injections without being overwhelmed. Needles still hurt a little as they went in. This is par for the course for anybody with a nervous system. Still, an injection right next to my eye was not my idea of a good time. I held my breath, stiffened up my muscles and waited for the small piece of material to be extracted. Phew, that's done. And it turned out to be benign and went away on its own.

Kidneys and Liver

Remember the nurse who said the body's ability to heal after illness is truly phenomenal? I have discovered this myself. As a consequence of GVHD my readings were not always perfect, especially for the liver, and the Prednisolone messed big time with my blood sugar levels and bone density. However, by late 2017 my kidney, liver and vitamin D levels returned to normal, and the high iron level slowly came down naturally. I should make a disclaimer here. The sepsis and ICU sojourn led to the kidney damage, and GVHD had also affected them, resulting in the actual function equating to only one kidney, not two. My kidneys were working at half-pace. This scared me until I realised one kidney is all that is required to live a healthy life. Evolution has provided us with an heir and a spare. How come we didn't end up with two brains, two hearts or two bladders I wondered?

Fred's appendix plays up

It was now Fred's turn to undergo another Medicare-funded medical intervention, a two-day hospital stay for an affliction usually experienced by much younger patients. During a visit to Sydney, Fred experienced pain in the region of his appendix. A trip to the excellent Emergency Department at St Vincent's Hospital indicated an issue which needed monitoring – possible appendicitis. Sure enough, the pain level ratcheted up a few weeks later so he went back to our home base, The Alfred naturally, for a midnight session of keyhole surgery. The operation was a success with no complications. Fred felt some discomfort for a few days. It was especially painful when he walked but painkillers helped with that. I wished my GVHD could be fixed with some quick keyhole surgery.

Now it's my liver

Fast forward to the beginning of 2018 and good news came my way. Professor Curtis took a look at my blood levels and reams of numbers relating to the health of my kidneys and liver. He declared them to be excellent; so excellent in fact that he said I was just like Benjamin Button – getting younger rather than older. I was so happy to hear this. We decided to stop the immunosuppressant drugs. My hope level ratcheted up. How good would a future be without the drugs?

My happiness did not last. Some not so good readings and test results were on the horizon.

At my next appointment in July it was clear the stronger donor cells had not given up their day (and night) job of taking over my body. GVHD symptoms such as mouth ulcers, sore, dry, itchy eyes and low energy were obvious (fortunately I didn't have skin rashes). What was happening inside my body was more of a worry. Professor Curtis looked at the numbers again and declared that although my kidneys were fine, my liver had gone haywire!

Back onto the Prednisolone, Tacrolimus and Valaciclovir. My first words on hearing this were – Please, please, do I have to stay on the Prednisolone for long? I don't want to deal with diabetes again. I reduced my consumption of carrot cakes, chocolate and ice cream, which made me feel deprived as I really craved sugar. I monitored my blood glucose level with the usual ouch factor finger prick tests first thing in the morning. At 8, it was slightly higher than normal and then varied from 6.7 to 12. Over the next two months things settled down, going back to near-normal as the Prednisolone dose was reduced. I was still reading as pre-diabetic but managing to avoid giving myself insulin injections. What a relief. I continued my regular blood tests and Professor Curtis adjusted the drug levels.

Time for a few more tests – eyes and bowel. I always worried a little beforehand. An eye examination, covered by Medicare, showed no sign of glaucoma or cataracts. One eye was stronger, the other weaker than the previous test so I needed new glasses. I told the optometrist I occasionally experienced jagged lightning flashes in my eyes which lasted for around ten minutes. Very space-age. She explained it was probably a migraine aura and usually wasn't serious. I did the free bowel cancer test which came in the mail. It is an excellent initiative compliments of the Federal Government. The test came out negative so all good there. Negative is the new positive.

One thing was for sure. I now knew more about my body than most people on the planet know about theirs; every physical aspect from top to toe had been analysed and discussed, not by choice but by necessity.

Lungs

October 2018. More not-so-good readings and test results to deal with. A serious virus similar to the flu went around and Fred and I both caught it. I lay in bed and waited for the debilitating symptoms to subside. Oddly, I did not have a fever or aches and pains. Just a feeling of malaise, lack of appetite and lack of energy. I was flat emotionally too; in fact I lacked hope. Fred saw the doctor. His virus turned into bronchitis but he made quite a quick recovery. I saw my local GP. An X-ray showed a dark patch on my left lung, as did a second X-ray. I now worried that I had lung cancer and fantasised about the bad cells clogging up my lungs until I finally suffocated and died. I was wrong. Because of my lowered immunity I scored a mild dose of bronchopneumonia, an infection which affects the air passages that feed air into the lungs. This was the likely cause of the lung shadow.

I checked out Dr Google and now worried I had new, serious lung problems. I was so sick of being sick. I spent the next two weeks in quite a depressed state. I didn't feel like doing anything except hanging around the house or sleeping and lost interest in food, writing and gardening.

I awaited the next blood test with trepidation. The test showed my liver had deteriorated and the kidneys were affected too. Time to up the Prednisolone dosage yet again. I tried to take control of my destiny in regards to possible insulin injections by asking if there were drugs which can lower BGL levels. Yes, there were. I now took quite a cocktail of drugs. The pneumonia improved and the sugar levels were lower again. I gave my donor cells a little talking to and waited for my hard-working liver to recover. Go for it liver, you are a top organ, a special organ. I need you to be healthy. You can do it.

My next blood test stripped away the veneer of courage I had cultivated so carefully regarding needles. As sometimes happens, the nurse in blood collection missed the vein by a fraction of a millimetre. Pain followed. It hurt. I whimpered then burst into tears. She ended up taking the blood from my hand instead. That hurt too. Inevitably, the same nurse took my blood again at my next visit. We eyed each other off as she checked me into room two. I parked myself on the familiar fat blue chair with the big wide arms, pulled up the sleeve of my shirt and closed my eyes tight. She applied the tourniquet and gently slid the needle into the crook of my arm. This time I breathed a sigh of relief. She did a great job. The experience was totally painless.

A further blood test showed a big improvement in liver function. The test also showed a big drop in kidney function, along with a low level of magnesium, not surprising given the toll of the pneumonia on my body. Professor Curtis made more adjustments to the drug dosage. One of the blood sugar control drugs which had made me nauseous and given me diarrhoea was eliminated. By the end of November my kidney function came back to near normal, if you count only having the functional equivalent of one kidney as normal. The liver kept improving, however vitamin D levels were now low.

What an endless emotional (and physical) roller coaster ride! If only it would stop so I could get off for a while and rest.

And what about my initial dodgy lung X-ray results I hear you ask? I didn't have any shortness of breath, persistent cough or excess phlegm which was a great sign. My GP naturally recommended further X-rays. It was not cancer, thank goodness, but the scans did indicate issues. A CT scan was requested. It looked into the lungs in more detail, in slices. The report promptly came back, in doctor speak of course. The CT appearances were consistent with mild changes of chronic interstitial lung disease... and some low grade changes of traction bronchiectasis. There was a broad differential diagnosis for this appearance including fibrosing alveolitis most commonly. No chest infection or congestive heart failure was diagnosed and my adrenal glands were of normal size so that was something positive to cling to. What the hell? Chronic lung disease? Time for another medical lesson. I needed to find out more about what the report revealed. The reassuring words mild and low grade did not sink in.

I had a lung condition which caused inflammation and scar tissue, irreversible dilation of the bronchi and bronchioles which are the passages which bring air into the lungs plus some inflammation and scarring of the walls of the tiny air sacs in the lungs. Professor Curtis said the respiratory changes were most likely a side effect of GVHD. I later read chemo can also cause lung issues. Smoking between the ages of fourteen and twenty-four would not have helped either. Bloody hell! What next. If phlegm gathered in my lungs I would have to hang upside down like a fruit bat to clear it. On the other hand I had a new excuse for not doing something as the cancer excuse was starting to wear thin. Sorry, I can't do any cooking, or wash the dishes for that matter. Don't you know I have lung disease?

The next blood test showed my kidneys had improved. The liver was still in dodgy territory. I made a plan. I aimed to get off the steroids merry go round.

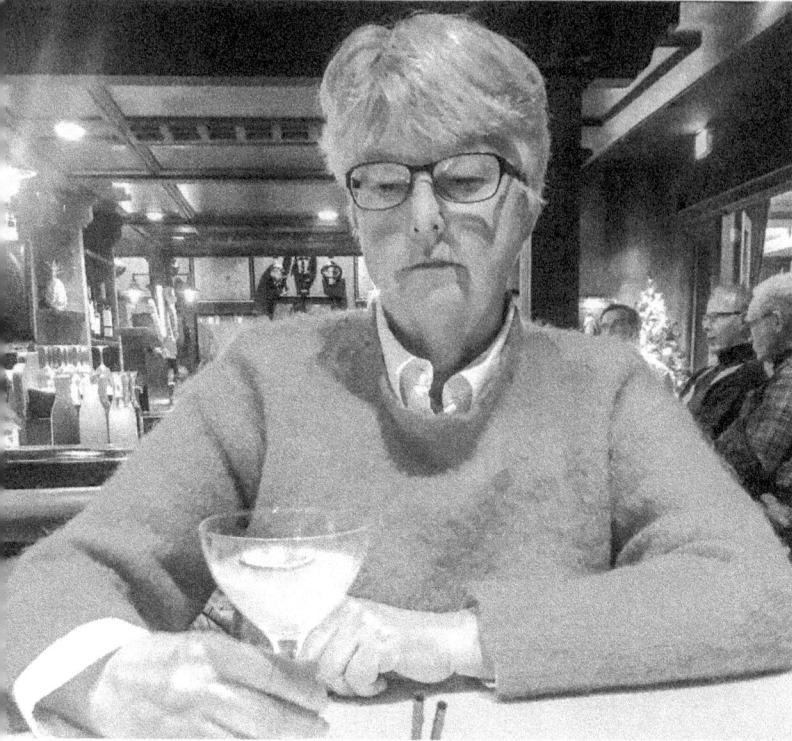

Cocktail hour wearing a favourite jumper knitted by Mum.

Then a strange thing happened. Once more my energy levels improved, the neurosis reduced and a degree of contentment returned. I gardened again, cleaned up the house like a domestic goddess and travelled into town. Fred retired after forty-four years in the workforce. We moved out of the inner city flat and into a new phase in our lives. The time had come to live exclusively in the country. Good friends Tim and Ronda visited over Christmas/New Year and we entertained guests for lunch. Fred cooked up a storm; everything from dry fried fish curries to roast chicken to spaghetti vongole. I was now living in the top paddock, that's for sure. I drank sparkling concoctions and gin and tonics most nights after 5pm, ate ice cream with my summer raspberries (I'm into seasonality) and managed to forget that my days might be even more numbered.

And still it went on...

I had health homework to do after the fourth Late Effects Clinic in November 2018. In January I had a mammogram. It is always fun to have your breasts flattened out like a pancake. All good; no breast cancer issues to deal with. Next, an uncomfortable but necessary Pap smear test. Cervix all good too.

I had plenty more follow up appointments at The Alfred. A talk with the osteoporosis specialist left me with lots to contemplate. The bone health of my hips was satisfactory but my spine had lost bone density as a side effect of the Prednisolone. I was instructed to do weight bearing exercises, so Fred and I joined the local council gym. We started off slowly. I managed to get through all the exercises and especially liked the treadmill because it had an inbuilt TV with the channel turned to fuzzy old black and white English movies. I noticed how many of the machines displayed little illustrations of men (not women) and what part of their body was being converted to buffness. I tried not to look sideways at all the toned young bodies or compare them to my chubby shape and flabby tummy.

Although I wanted to live in denial, the endocrinologist told me I was again classified as diabetic, thanks to the steroids, and had to take a BGL reading before breakfast and before dinner. I was told sugar consumption must be reduced. Luckily I was not addicted to soft drinks but it should be obvious to you by now that I am rather fond of anything sweet. Fred often came in and asked if I had checked my BGL level. I told him I was scared the level would be too high. I will do it tomorrow. I promise. OK, I give in. I'll do it now.

I like to put things off. I recall a check-up where Professor Curtis, who had an intern sitting in, asked me to describe the function of the three drugs I was taking. I failed the test. I could not describe them with any accuracy which was crazy as I had been taking them for months and details about all my drugs were listed on a special sheet. I had not made the effort for two reasons. I trusted my doctor to prescribe the right stuff and I had run out of energy to learn how these concoctions worked, and their side effects. It is too easy to leave everything to your doctor. Like Ingrid Bergman said in the movie *Casablanca*, 'You have to think for both of us. For all of us.'

Next, a visit to The Alfred's lung specialist for a lung function test. Even with my dodgy lungs the latest test surprisingly showed an improvement over the one undertaken prior to my transplant. I saw Professor Curtis early in March 2019. My kidney and liver function again showed an improvement, so we reduced the steroids slowly from 10mg daily to a low dose of 5mg. Those organs were up and down like a yoyo. Snappy graphs on the computer assisted the Professor in keeping track. The latest bone density tests, called DEXA, now showed some bone loss both in the spine and hips but a low risk of fracture. I supposed I should have been thankful for small mercies. I was still breathing so that was a bonus.

Time to meet with The Alfred's diabetes educator. I showed her a table of blood glucose readings over the previous week. Too high. A daily insulin injection to reduce the levels again became inevitable as the dietary changes on their own were not working. Must have been those Tim Tams I ate. My morning routine commenced with the usual finger prick blood test. I then took all the usual prescribed tablets and vitamins and gave myself the usual injection of insulin in the tummy. I was an old hand at this procedure now. Left-hand side one day, right-hand side the next. I shook the pen to mix the white liquid, screwed on the needle and did a little test to make sure it flowed properly. Holding my breath and tensing up, I administered the correct dosage, observing the needle breaking the skin and feeling the familiar small rush of anxiety. The BGL levels came down.

One week in, unwanted feelings overwhelmed me, similar to three years before, the last time I had to inject insulin. Feelings of dread, slight nausea, lack of energy, lack of appetite, a slight cough, the feeling of an oncoming cold that didn't turn into anything. And my heart rate was at the high end of normal at 100 beats per minute. Was I starting to crack up again? Thoughts of falling off the perch preoccupied me. Maybe I needed some serotonin enhancement. Was I transforming into a medical narcissist? Once more my body was betraying me.

EIGHT

—————

Why Me?

Initially I didn't think, Why have I developed cancer? But inevitably my mind did wander down that path over the past nine years. AML is thought to result from damage to one or more of the genes that normally control blood cell development. What causes this damage? Risk factors include: exposure to very high doses of radiation, either accidentally (nuclear accident) or therapeutically (in cancer treatment); industrial chemicals like benzene, which occurs naturally in crude oil, over a long period; pesticides, paint strippers and certain cleaning products; certain types of chemotherapy to treat other cancers; having a genetic syndrome; cancer-causing substances in tobacco smoke; general environmental toxins; getting older. So many things I have been exposed to, could it have been one of them?

Cigarette Smoke and other chemicals?

I was exposed to my father's second-hand cigarette and cigar smoke for eighteen years and I was a pack-a-day smoker for ten years from the young age of fourteen. I started off on Alpine Menthols to reduce the harshness of cigarette smoke and to cool the throat, and followed up with Marlboro Reds (the macho Marlboro Man was a big deal but I don't recall any Marlboro Women), heavy duty filter-less Camels because a boyfriend smoked them, or Sobranie Cocktail cigarettes for the girly colours and classy gold filter.

I lived on an orchard in the 1960s where Dad used a multitude of pesticides in order to produce the perfectly formed fruit demanded by the cannery. I regularly coloured my hair and developed hundreds of photographs in a darkroom without gloves or proper ventilation. I used a utility with a diesel engine for my gardening business and drove it long distances.

Did any of these factors increase my risk of cancer? Did I get sick because of the life choices I made? Looking back I could have made even worse choices – consuming lots of junk food and soft drinks, continuing smoking, sun tanning every day without sunscreen...

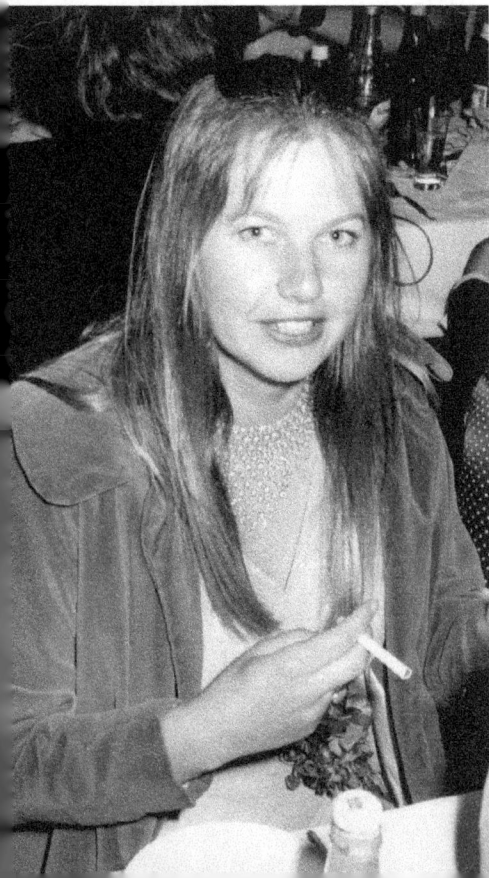

La Trobe University Ball 1974,
Marlboro Reds at the ready.

No Tonsils?

Recently I came across articles which made me think the early removal of my tonsils and catching measles as a child may be connected to my cancer. In addition to leading to hospitalisation and needle phobia, both events had a negative impact on my immune system in ways I did not fully grasp until now. The tonsils, which are a set of lymphoid organs, play a specialised role as a first line of defence against bacterial and viral infections. They can even make T cells. Tonsillectomy is associated with an increased risk for diseases of the upper respiratory tract such as asthma, influenza, pneumonia and chronic bronchitis.

When childhood illnesses such as colds or stomach bugs appear, the immune system knows to attack those germs when they try to invade again. Two new studies in The Netherlands have found the measles virus kills the memory cells that make antibodies. This apparently leaves the child vulnerable to catching other infectious diseases for several years after the measles. So my immune system received a double whammy in childhood. Looking back, apart from contracting pneumonia after the measles, I was often sick with ear infections, colds and the flu. There is even a comment in a primary school report noting that I had missed many days of school. It also makes me wonder if my lack of immunity carried on into adulthood, making my body vulnerable to the growth of abnormal cells.

Environmental factors
– dieldrin and other pesticide exposure

Late in 2018 a news item gave me an unexpected start, a moment of recognition. A cluster of young people had died, mainly of blood-related cancers including AML, on Victoria's Bellarine Peninsula. Scores of others had experienced similar illnesses leading to suspicions that an environmental cause was behind this cluster.

The broad-spectrum pesticide dieldrin was widely used by potato farmers in the district in the past. The United States EPA prohibited its manufacture in 1974 however dieldrin was only banned in Australia in 1987 after beef exported to the US and Japan tested positive for excessive levels. This led to two hundred Bellarine Peninsula farms being quarantined. Dieldrin is a form of synthetic organochlorine pesticide from the same family as DDT, heptachlor, aldrin and chlordane. According to a report by the University of Hertfordshire it is a neurotoxin and probably a mutagen which is highly toxic to mammals and remains in the soil for decades.

My father regularly used dieldrin on our orchard in the 1960s and 70s, as did many fruit farmers in the district. Rows of beautiful apricot trees pruned to a vase shape formed our backyard and Dad also grew peaches and pears on our irrigated forty acre plot. We consumed fresh and bottled fruit year round. Being a farmer was not easy. Dad had to contend with hailstorms, frosts, competition from the European Common Market and South African growers and the demands of the cannery. The fruit had to be of perfect size and blemish free. Dad told me he hated spraying the industrial quantities of chemicals he used to kill insects such as scale, codling moth or to counteract brown rot. He was certainly diligent when applying the chemical soup. He always wore top to

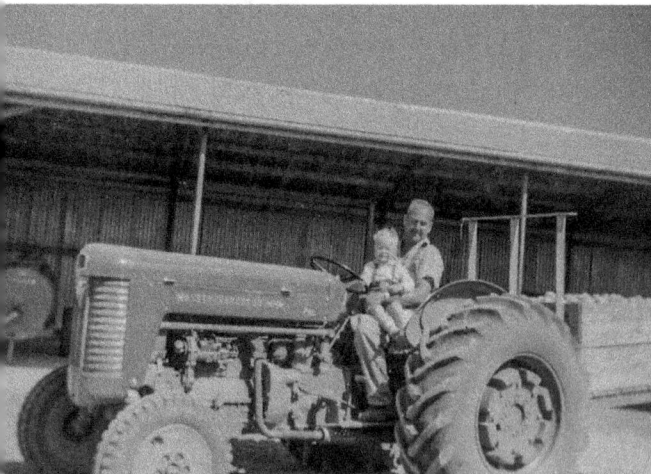

Dad and John. Note the spray tank on the left.

toe protective gear including a mackintosh and face mask. The red spray pump he towed behind the tractor expelled a vast toxic mist which wafted everywhere. Our drinking water came via a big corrugated tank with the rainwater captured from the roof of our house. Chemical residue no doubt contaminated the entire roof after Dad sprayed the fruit trees. It is difficult to know what ended up in an innocent-looking glass of water.

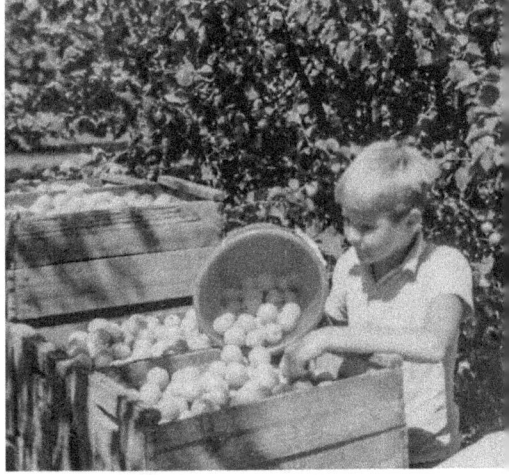

Peter picking apricots 1967.

My brother John recalls watching, from his primary school, a crop duster spraying nearby fruit trees. The seat he sat on became wet with spray. He also remembers a neighbour spraying left over DDT around his farm. Shortly afterwards he found dead magpies and swore never to use it again. The inside of our home received the DDT treatment too; compliments of products such as Shelltox which mum would liberally spray around using a bicycle pump type apparatus. As the advertising proudly declared, its DDT content remains deadly for months.

Dieldrin was not the only chemical Dad applied. I came across a neat bright yellow cardboard calculator which helped him apply the correct amount of carbendazim fungicide, commercially known as Bavastin, a potion which is highly toxic to earthworms. Dad also used another organochlorine insecticide, Malathion, which is still on the market. It is highly toxic to bees.

Do an internet search on the science behind these products; it is scary stuff. Nice little earners for the chemical companies but at what cost? Paul Hermann Müller was awarded the Nobel Prize in Physiology or Medicine 1948 for his discovery of the high efficiency of DDT as a contact poison against several arthropods. DDT turned out to be double edged sword; it saved many people from diseases such as malaria. It also became a serious environmental toxin.

I cannot prove it of course, however there may be a connection between the chemicals I was exposed to as a child and my AML. I wonder if a blood test would detect any pesticide residues in my blood or urine. Given the numerous blood transfusions I have undergone and the massive changes to my blood brought about by the stem cell transplant the answer would probably be no.

I support local farmers and buy organic local food whenever possible including pasture fed eggs and vegetables such as garlic, corn and potatoes. There are regular farmers markets and suppliers in most nearby towns and lately kind locals have been dropping off their delicious excess produce outside the general store, including tomatoes and blood oranges. I reciprocated with Italian parsley which grows like a forest in my garden. Organic foods and green cleaning products can also be found in our supermarkets. To me it is a no brainer even though it costs a bit more.

Cancer is everywhere, and everyone has to deal with it, and the possibility of death, in their own way. It is a club with millions of members; albeit a club that no-one asks to join. In the years before and since my diagnosis a number of family and friends have coped with all kinds of cancer, from breast to prostate, cervical to bowel, blood and lung. While some have died, many have lived on. Some chose the alternative route including medical marijuana (sounds like a plan), vitamin C infusions, a vegan diet, meditation, yoga and visits to psychics; others took the medical option or a combination of both. Some were optimists and others not so much. Is there any connection between their positivity or negativity and cancer survival rates? The outcome is dependent on so many factors. You may be the most positive person in town, have the best organic diet, never smoked or consumed alcohol, taken measures to reduce stress, exercise regularly and still get sick. You might be constantly stressed out; smoke two packs a day and live to ninety-eight. It's a crapshoot.

I often read that small amounts of a particular pesticide, herbicides such as glyphosate or food additives will not be harmful to health. Like Jane Goodall I cannot believe that applying toxins to our food is a good idea. Where is the research which investigates if and how a *combination* of these laboratory chemicals affects us? Has it gone into the too hard basket? At this stage I have no idea if any of the chemicals I have been exposed to in my life had a direct effect on my cancer diagnosis however I suspect there is a connection. A spin of the wheel, a drop or two of pesticide and some poorly functioning cells and yes, come on down, you have cancer. Like many cancer patients, I suspect, I have wasted too much time thinking about the what ifs. Hindsight is a wonderful thing but it didn't cure my cancer and thinking about what I shouldn't have done in the past won't help me in the future.

Nevertheless an awareness of the dangers of chemicals is not a bad thing but further research needs to be done on the connection between pesticides and leukaemia. There could be a Nobel Prize in it.

NINE

——

It's all in the mind

The cure nearly killed me

Although there have been amusing and even enjoyable aspects to my cancer journey, the experience did have a huge psychological impact. I ran the gamut of emotions – fear, amusement, resignation, numbness, curiosity, anger, sadness. It was intense. As I have detailed in *Who am I?*, this impact was exacerbated by the excess baggage I carried stemming from medical incidents in childhood. To top it off, many challenging life events happened as I struggled to recover. I was given assistance from the hospital with the emotional side to some extent and saw their therapist twice. Although I am a resilient person, I certainly needed further help to deal with the stresses I faced, stresses that did not end when I left hospital. Somehow I found the inner resources to manage my fears because I had no alternative if I wanted to survive, but everyone's needs are different. The important thing is to get suitable help if and when you need it.

I read somewhere that looking forward to the future is a crucial element of a satisfying life – travel, time with family, creating a vegie patch, a better job or the next game of football. True. Serious illness can take away your hope. You don't know if you have a future.

The three plus weeks spent in ICU were especially surreal; a real test of my emotional stability. According to Dr Raymond Raper, intensivist and president of the College of Intensive Care Medicine, intensive care is awful, uncomfortable, invasive and undignified and it's not an ordeal you should put anybody through unless you can offer a reasonable prospect of getting back to a good quality of life.* Dr Raper also emphasised that the assessment of what constitutes a good quality of life is that of the patient. Every person who has been in ICU should be offered therapy. After all, they have usually been through a traumatic near-death experience.

Seeing a therapist outside of the hospital certainly helped address my plunges into anxiety. And being able to express my feelings to Fred and asking for his advice was an essential element in my recovery.

Time to express some feelings

One memorable night in ICU, as the nurse sat politely across from us, Fred and I quietly cried and talked together. He was my rock. There to provide whatever support he could, both emotionally and physically 24/7. For weeks he had been spending hours every day at the hospital, in addition to working full-time. He had been through a hell of a lot and needed support too. When your loved one is close to dying you are way out of your depth. It was a new experience for both of

---

* Kate Aubusson. https://www.smh.com.au/national/covid-19-robbed-tom-of-oxygen-mechanical-breaths-and-whispered-words-brought-him-back-20200508-p54ran.html

us. It was an awful test for him, and he was suffering. He told me later that he never felt resentful of my helplessness and the new demands being placed on him. If the situation had been reversed I'm not sure I would have been capable of such constant support.

Anxiety in ICU

One morning in ICU, after I had emerged from my coma, extreme agitation set in. This seemed to come out of the blue. It was not like me to experience this level of angst, even in hospital. Whether I was suddenly comprehending the enormity of my experience or it was the effect of the drugs I was being given I don't know, but I became really frightened. Suddenly I had had enough and my brain snapped. I had no idea what the time was. I panicked. Where was Fred? I had to ring him. Help me! Get me out of here. Please. Please, I yelled down the phone in my still scratchy voice. He told me later he felt so sad and helpless when he heard me say this. Thankfully he soon arrived. I was so relieved to see him.

Imagining the end

I did not have a Hickman inserted while in ICU, just cannulas here, there and everywhere, including in my groin. Just an over-medicated pin cushion. Lying in bed with tubes hanging out left and right precluded the usual tossing and turning that happens during a normal night's sleep. It seemed to focus the mind and provided the opportunity for more fantasising. I could not take much more of this. I had reached the end of my rope.

I pictured how to do it.

Option 1: Somehow stockpile a selection of the myriad of drugs being pumped into me. That wouldn't work, even though I was often asked if I was in pain and could get a Panadol or two to store under my pillow. The nurse generally compounded the drugs into a powder with a pestle and mortar. (Which is the pestle and which is the mortar I wondered?) I decided it would be impossible to secretly get hold of a large enough caché of tablets.

Option 2: Will myself to expire using my superior mental powers. That wouldn't work either, given my mental powers were now inferior to Superman's or even an ordinary mortal.

Option 3: Stop breathing. No go. The nurse would revive me and I could only hold my breath for a short time anyway. It looked like I had to keeping on living.

Option 4: Ask the doctors if they could help out. That wasn't going to fly. Remember the Hippocratic Oath?

ICU was the last place I could bump myself off, seeing the whole aim of the place was to keep me alive.

ICU played tricks with my mind

All the staff seemed to float or mince around the place. My brain was still scrambled. Photographs of Gus the cat, our friendly user, sleeping on the ironing board; artist and good friend David who faced severe health issues of his own, including prostate cancer; our American buddies Jim and Paulette and our garden had made their way from 7 East and were now pinned to the notice board in my room.

One day in my mind's eye the board had totally disappeared. At other times I could not read the time on the wall clock. Half the hands were gone or appear to be back to front. Time took on a new meaning. I did not know what day it was, let alone what time it was. My poor brain did not work properly.

In my addled imagination the muscle-bound man in the room next to me happened to be a big-time central European criminal hiding out from his enemies in the ICU. It surprised me no-one else saw he was in there under false pretences. Look, he was able to walk around and maybe even leave the hospital under his own steam. What I didn't see was him projectile vomiting all over the place one day. Fred described it in some detail to me later.

Fear of needles subsided

By 27 December 2012, I had undergone a mind-boggling twenty-two blood tests outside of my hospitalisations (and made twelve visits to the doctor). If I had been told when I first went into hospital in March that I would have this many blood tests in a three-month time period I would not have made it past the front door. One positive aspect of this was my terror of needles had now markedly decreased. I didn't have the spare energy to generate that much trepidation. And, I happened to have a Hickman to make life easier and avoid needle punctures.

Fears

A few months later I attend an AML support group. We shared our survivor stories in a round table over coffee and cakes. I learned how badly GVHD had affected some of the attendees and left for home feeling quite depressed and worried about my future. By now the whole AML experience had left me with some symptoms of post-traumatic stress, (remnants of which I still experience). Fred bore the brunt of my anxiety, my constant looking out for danger, real or imagined. I worried about driving my car and turned into an annoying front seat driver. Watch out! I viewed other drivers as mindless morons, a threat to my life. When Fred bumped into me or made a sudden loud sound, I jumped or screamed and ended up giving him a fright. It was hard to relax. Walking down any stairs made me feel unsteady. Walking on a flat surface was tiring. Walking upstairs was even more tiring.

I wondered if I would ever feel normal again.

Death of my mother

Aside from cancer, life did go on with its ups and downs. More than one journalist has stated the obvious in magazine and newspaper articles – serious illness, being unable to work, moving house, financial pressures and getting married can all be high stress life events. Add the death of a parent to the mix in the same year and you have a full hand; a royal flush of challenging circumstances. My mother died on 11 November 2012. She was 86.

She had a small stroke in September and by early October another stroke had put her back in hospital. My energy was down after the transplant, so even visiting the hospital to see her was an exhausting excursion. I worried about what I could do to help her. Mum would stay in bed and now refused to eat the pureed food.

'Mum, you have to eat,' I said.

'You didn't want to eat the hospital food,' she replied. Well, that was true but still a tricky answer on her part. The situation was somewhat different.

Mum had been living with my brother John but after a few weeks it became clear she was not coming back home. The next step would be the nursing home. Even though I was still frail I managed to drag myself around to see her fairly regularly in hospital.

I certainly regretted keeping Mum away from my hospital bed in the early stage of my hospitalisation. That is said from the perspective of relative wellness. The reality was I was feeling so ill at the time I had no other option.

At her hospital bed I told Mum how much I loved her and thanked her for the love and care she gave me and my brothers. By this stage Mum was already moving away from us. She looked pale and a bit spaced out as she smiled at me but I am sure she heard me. On that last night we all kissed her and sadly said goodbye. I felt so despondent. Not long after we arrived home the phone call came to say she had died. I wish I had stayed on but Mum waited until we all left the room to make her final move.

Mum had organised a pre-paid funeral. All we had to do was organise the flowers, sandwiches, music and photos for a slide show. I did not cry at the funeral although I wanted to. My feelings had been pushed down too far after coping with own my illness. Mum had chosen her time to leave. She told me not to make grieving a long term project which gave me some solace. I'm glad she did not have to face one of her children dying before her.

Heart surgery

Ten months after Mum died Fred would unwittingly compete with me for the most challenging medical affliction award – major heart surgery. It was a strange thing. I discovered when you are subjected to one stressful event after another you become a little punch drunk. You think you can't take it anymore. You discover that somehow you can take it. The next issue becomes another resilience test. Join the queue.

Something else to deal with. It was serious but you keep coping – but it all adds up.

Ten months after my transplant we travelled to Europe for five weeks, staying at marvellous bed and breakfasts from The Netherlands to France and Italy. After we arrived back home Fred told me he had experienced chest pains on the return flight which he interpreted as indigestion. The pains did not persist and the Qantas A380, crew and passengers did not have to divert to the nearest Middle East airport. That would have been something to write home about. However he had actually experienced a minor heart attack.

A few weeks later he had another attack. This time, being at work at Monash University which is up the road from the Monash Medical Centre, help was immediately at hand. Diagnosis – atherosclerosis (narrowing of the arteries due to a build-up of plaque).

The short-term solution was to unblock an artery with a stent. This was done. Some months later another solution offered a longer-term benefit – heart surgery or to use the correct medical term coronary artery bypass graft. Following the recommendation of his specialist Fred decided to go for it.

This was scary stuff, and not the first experience I had had of this disease. The same affliction led to the premature death of my father at sixty-two.

Once more Fred and I put our faith in Australia's public health system and once more it came up trumps. Heart bypass is not for the faint hearted (no pun intended), even if it is done by an experienced team of surgeons. On 20 January 2014 Fred was admitted to the Monash Medical Centre. He was understandably anxious. He spent the entire afternoon in surgery.

Before he was wheeled into the operating theatre I knew there was a chance this would be the last time I saw him but I did not expend too much energy dwelling on this. The numbers were in his favour as the risk of death after this operation is only 1-2%. Amazing when you learn about what is done.

The operation was successful. Happy, happy days.

It was now my turn to play nurse, cook and be personal assistant. My energy levels were still low but it was a task I happily took on. It was a relief that Fred had made it through the surgery. Although he was not pleased about it, Fred was made to walk around the ward two days after the operation and came home a few days after that. The recovery was not easy and he felt pretty awful for some time but slowly he began to heal. I sent emails around to keep our friends and family in the loop, like Fred had done for me. In one I noted: We must both be in the go hard or go home category in regards to health issues. Thank goodness there are medical people around us to help us.

Underestimating the emotional effect of treatment

From March 2014 I felt well enough to take a casual job working front-of-house as a team leader at a local theatre. I did this for a few months. I had done this work in the past so the tasks were familiar. But I didn't take my general level of anxiety and lowered energy level into account. At first I secretly became terrified of a whole range of things, driving to the venue, making a mistake setting up the bar, instructing the ushers or balancing the takings at the end of the night. Nevertheless I managed to get through each shift without major stuff-ups and the work became easier over time.

Stress and illness

Researchers are finding increasing evidence that we store trauma such as being abused as a child (or being held down on the operating table?) in our body and this trauma can alter the way our brain works, putting us permanently on high alert and affecting the immune system. According to researchers at Yale University, childhood trauma can increase the risk of inflammation and manifest later in diseases such as cancer.

I asked Professor Curtis if he thought there was a *direct* link between chronic stress and cancer. He replied, If stress causes cancer we would all have the disease. That made me think. Some studies indicate that stress does cause cancer or increases someone's risk; others have shown no connection.

Self-assurance

When I was around nine-years-old I had a lucky escape from an abuser who crossed my path. One of my teachers attempted to molest me at his house but I courageously walked straight out the door, trekked four long miles home and told Mum what had happened. She believed me without question. Dad immediately confronted the teacher and threatened to kill him if he even came near me again. I am so grateful my parents stepped in to protect me, even if Dad was a little heavy-handed. This experience, although disturbing, helped me to deal with the vicissitudes of life, including my cancer. I knew when faced with a crisis I had the support of my parents.

It laid the foundation for developing a strong sense of self-assurance. I knew I had the ability, especially with support, to take on challenges and somehow find a way to deal with whatever confronted me. Self-assurance had a key role to play.

Upbringing and the impact on the development of self

Although my parents expected me to do well at school and had strong ideas of right and wrong behaviour, they did not micro-manage day to day. I am so glad they let me free range on the weekends. I was happy to mess about at home or go fishing, ride my bike or swim in the main irrigation channel with my girlfriends – totally unsupervised. Mum's only rules were – don't mess around with the fruit pickers and; – make sure you are home for dinner.

Even though I had parents who loved and supported me and I didn't lack self-confidence, I still carried stresses from my past, compounded by having to deal with ongoing medical issues and confronting my own mortality. I needed help.

Get help

Cancer can have a huge impact on you and the people around you, not just physically but psychologically as well. The psychological impact can stay with you and emerge at times when you least expect it.

After my traumas injecting insulin I experienced another period of debilitating anxiety which was out of character and severely impacted on my ability to function. Fred and I discussed getting professional assistance. Our friend, Dr Russ Harris, knew a doctor who specialised in childhood medical trauma and hypnotherapy. Fred described my condition so accurately over the phone that she thought he must be a medical professional himself. As a general rule she did not treat adults but agreed to see me as I was an intriguing example of how a stressful childhood experience can manifest itself in the adult world.

So, I saw the doctor.

On my first visit to her welcoming rooms I hardly made it up the stairs. I was a quivering mess. After a chat she asked me to sit in the special patient's therapy chair. This chair felt good to sit in. I imagined a favourite colour, imagined injecting myself. The most frightening part? Actually, the needle going into my tummy did not usually hurt, only the idea of the needle. Just a little scratch little girl, just a little scratch.

As you know, I experienced a double whammy as a child – being forcibly held down on the operating table during the tonsillectomy and then suffering the intense pain of penicillin injections in the backside a few years later. The therapist believes, as I do, that these experiences can change a person for life because of potential damage to the developing brain. Vaccines for diseases such as tuberculosis may possibly have saved my life but avoiding blood tests for diseases such as leukaemia nearly killed me.

The therapist asked me to visualise being in a movie theatre, firstly sitting watching myself injecting, then watching from the projection room and being in the film injecting. In my mind I could not make the picture go into reverse, with the needle coming out and finishing at the start of the procedure, when imagining it in black and white. But I could reverse it when visualising in colour. The mind is astonishing and mysterious.

A feeling of despondency grew, leading to an insight. What I needed most at the time of my tonsil operation was to be hugged, held, comforted and enveloped, with accurate advance warning of what I was about to experience and the opportunity to talk about how I was feeling after the operation. I needed to be taught some coping skills but I imagine my parents were themselves facing anxieties with their child undergoing an unpleasant medical procedure.

You've got to be dreaming

Looking back on the many days and nights spent lying in my hospital bed, one vital ingredient of a normal life was totally missing – the ability to sleep properly and the opportunity to dream during REM sleep. It is an issue which is difficult to resolve for a cancer patient. By necessity the hospital routine is the polar opposite of peaceful and yet sleep is so essential for recovery. A friend who had been through a similar experience compared it to Melbourne's Flinders Street Station. Nurses, specialists, cleaners, food delivery staff, social workers, blood testers, pharmacists – it's non-stop action all day.

Then the night-time routine kicks in. It is a lot quieter, but the nurses understandably like to have a chat at their stations. Vital signs need to be checked every two or four hours, especially temperature. Signs of fever are taken seriously because it indicates the immune system is trying to fight infection. At 4am taking blood from a Hickman isn't the most intrusive procedure. However, when blood pressure is being measured, the cuff stiffening and squeezing around my arm always felt uncomfortable. And the trolley the nurses used to transport all their equipment had the noisiest set of wheels. You could hear it coming a mile away. Those wheels needed to be padded with fur or something soft.

So, not enough time for dreaming.

I became somewhat narcoleptic in hospital, falling asleep whenever I could, day or night. I still never managed to dream. It took a long time to get back to a normal sleep routine. Even now any dream, which writer Bryce Courtney called a natural problem-solving gift if we choose to use it, is most welcome, especially that rare experience of defying gravity and floating about in space.

In one dream I visited the Professor for a check-up. I waited patiently for the results of my latest blood test, especially my BGL reading, but he wouldn't tell me anything at all. No analysis needed to interpret this dream – each time I have a check-up I worry just a little that I will have to face more bad news.

Since the AML I often dream about music, theatre and celebrities. I have spent time in dream world hanging out with U2's Bono at arena concerts, ('You're kept awake dreaming someone else's dream...' is an apt line from U2's song *Electrical Storm*), and Brian Ferry was the good-looking receptionist at the weird dream hotel I recently stayed at. One time I dreamt I was Shirley Bassey's personal assistant. My job was to look after her luxurious mink coat and pink designer handbag when she walked onto the stage. I asked one of the ladies in the audience to look after the coat which ended up being thrown on a table laden with cocktails. I put her handbag on the side of the stage. All of a sudden the event turned chaotic. The audience began wrestling each other and bodies were being hurled across the room, turning into projectiles in mid-air. Utter mayhem. Shirley sang two bars of her classic number *Goldfinger* but then exited the stage quick smart. I woke up at this stage, before she sacked me.

I used to work front of house at Hoyts Cinema Centre, a major cinema complex in Melbourne. Lately I have repeatedly dreamt about that cinema. The anxiety theme may be familiar to you – turning up without my uniform or underwear on; trying to seat a full house of patrons in the dark without my torch; needing to go to the toilet, opening the door only to find a tiny cupboard, a door leading nowhere or a room without any facilities; taking a step down the stairs which suddenly becomes a huge chasm or walking up the stairs which quickly turns into a rock climbing exercise.

Surprising connections can occur thanks to the cancer experience. I discovered that a childhood nightmare had a basis in real events. For years I dreamt about Dad driving our little Standard 8 over a bridge and I became scared as the car was washed away by floodwaters. Using the National Library of Australia's online search engine, Trove, to see what else I could discover about those days, I came across a newspaper article in the *Dandenong Journal*. A bridge which crossed Dandenong Creek along the side of the Luxton property, where Dad worked, was in a dangerous condition. The bridge was particularly unsafe at night as part of the protective railing was missing. Cars continually needed assistance when they became stuck in the flooded road. So I was possibly reliving a real experience of being rescued or the fear of being caught in the flood.

I still have dreams of water and floods. It is weird how getting cancer can indirectly make sense of past experiences. It is only a small thing, but I may not have made the connection between the dream and crossing the flooded bridge in real-life without the cancer. That was not something I expected as a side-effect.

Friends have their own story to tell

I've always thought that one of the worst things about cancer is that you seem to have nothing else in your life, you become the illness for a while; it's all everyone seems to talk about, the rest of life seems to stop, which of course it has to so you can focus on getting better.

– Fran (my business partner at Your Gardening Angels)

As well as having an impact on Fred, my illness had an effect on others in ways I wasn't always aware of. Fred and I regularly met up with other Xavier College staff members from the boarding house days. Over dinner, Sonya, the former head chef, was chatting with me about my book and the emotions she felt when seeing me unconscious in ICU. I never knew she spent three hours quietly sitting there. Her strong impression was that the energetic person she knew had disappeared, replaced by someone who was now a shell of a human being. The care shown by the ICU staff amazed her. David, her oldest cousin, who she was very close to, was diagnosed with AML at eighteen and passed away the day after celebrating his twenty-first birthday. This had a profound effect on Sonya and led to a decision which has saved many lives. She regularly donates blood at the local Blood Bank. She is O negative which is special as it means her blood can be given to any patient who needs a transfusion. She is a true quiet achiever who does not seek out recognition but deserves it in spades.

Manny, who is the same age as I am, is another friend who visited me in ICU. She told me she could not deal with the situation. She became so upset she had to leave the room. In 2015 Manny was diagnosed with early stage breast cancer but is now cured. I asked her how she handled the news of her illness. The moment of realisation as she was asked to wait in another room for the outcome of her mammogram was a shock but she needed to know the truth. Deciding on conventional treatment, she underwent thirty-six tiring rounds of radiation therapy. She chose not to have the eighteen double doses offered as she felt at her age it would have knocked her out. The support of her husband and daughter helped her recovery from this nevertheless debilitating regime. Manny does not have any firm ideas as to the trigger for her cancer. Did she use positive thinking? She tried hard to ditch negative thoughts and avoided interaction with relatives and friends who might bring her down. Like Sonya, helping others has become an important, in fact vital, part of her life. She has become a volunteer. Every week she visits residents at a nearby retirement home which gives her tremendous satisfaction. Gardening does that for me, in spades.

TEN

Becoming a Carer – Fred's thoughts

I asked Fred to write about being a Carer. Here is his experience:

Caring for someone with a life-threatening illness like cancer can be very challenging. In all probability it will be thrust upon you without warning. Your world can be turned upside down in a flash and I hope my ruminations will help you navigate these tricky waters. When Cathy was diagnosed with leukaemia, it was only a matter of hours before I felt quite overwhelmed. My first thought when her diagnosis was confirmed was that she might not survive. It was a total shock and surprise – something that had never entered my mind. I felt truly frightened at the reality of possibly losing her altogether. My feelings were pretty confused and I felt a strange mixture of disbelief, sadness, disorientation and even a little anger.

How was I going to cope? I soon realized unless I managed my feelings and the fear and uncertainty suddenly thrust upon me, I was not going to be able to care for her. I cried quite a bit that first day alone in our flat. What would I do if she did not survive? Could I spend the rest of my life without her? The important thing at this time was that no one told me it would be OK and that I should not feel so stunned and emotional. No one said be strong! That was a good thing as I did not at that point feel strong, just overwhelmed.

Over the coming few days, I began to get organised around what needed to be done, how to deal with my life now, finding a way to balance my full time job and being with Cathy, along with managing family, friends and communications. I suspect my event management experience kicked in, although I did feel quite fragile at times.

In order to truly help someone, particularly someone very close to you, what they need becomes paramount. That's not easy as all sorts of confronting things will happen over the course of the days, weeks and months. I did not, or tried not to, dwell on the what ifs. I wanted information about the disease and treatment but my focus became how to support my partner in what was now a real life and death moment. What did she need the most from me? I did not stop her from having any of the feelings she was having, whatever they were. Then I had to provide what she needed. Being available 24-hours a day, either in person or on the phone, was key, so she could contact me at any time. It was essential to give her the space to focus on herself and to keep everyone in the loop with what was happening.

Being honest as a caregiver is critical. In my opinion it is vital to not stifle or prevent your loved one from talking about their fears, the possibility of not surviving, and how awful the experience is. It is really awful. Use your judgement and your knowledge of your partner/family member to work out the best way to treat them. I knew platitudes like 'you will be fine' or 'don't talk like that' were generally not helpful with Cathy, which I am sure is the case with many people. Being able to reassure Cathy how I was managing my life throughout this period without her; that the bills were being paid, work was fine, I was getting enough sleep, and yes, the cat was being looked after was important information for her too. Occasionally I deferred telling her something that might worry her unduly. For example, our cat Gus disappeared for three days when Cathy was undergoing her first chemo in hospital. I did not tell her straight away even though I was worried he had been killed on the road or had run away. He did finally return as if nothing was wrong, and only then did I tell her of his adventure away from the flat.

One of the truly difficult aspects was how to engage with family and friends. Cathy made it clear she felt unable to see anyone after the first two days of treatment. She had no energy or capacity to deal directly with people needing to see her and relate to her or ask her questions. She could not even talk much of the time. Some patients may say they are happy to see and speak to friends and family but the reality is it's exhausting and possibly unhelpful to their recovery, so you may need to intervene. As Cathy's principal carer, I felt I had to find a way to manage all of this direct and indirect communication. In order to deal with it, I recalled what an American friend had done during his wife's long stay in a Los Angeles ICU on the brink of death from a severe lung disease. With family and friends spread all over the USA, and a few internationally, he created an email group list, and every couple of days he sent an email with the latest information. This had the effect of everyone feeling they were in the loop and engaged with the process. It reduced the number of individual phone calls required to keep people informed. I decided to do the same. Each evening I would email the updates and progress to around fifty friends and family. Emailing everyone daily was a good way for me to talk about each day's events and feel positive when things were going well, but not ignore the reality when things were not great.

I would take any messages and replies to the emails into the hospital for Cathy to read. This helped me too. I did not have to repeat things endlessly over the phone, which can be quite debilitating, and provided me with a way of literally downloading the day's events.

I did phone Cathy's mum most days with a regular update. I had proposed this directly to her when I had met with the family about Cathy requesting no visits until she felt stronger. The issue of no visits can be quite a vexed one. Some patients, I am sure, encourage visits from family and friends. Others will find this too exhausting and demanding. I felt it was essential to establish what she needed, and in consultation with her, provide the safest and least stressful environment for her treatment and recovery.

Being quietly present can be a challenge. I realized that sitting with Cathy and not necessarily talking was crucial. I also made sure to ask her what she needed. Initially, when it was permitted, some tasty non-hospital food was a godsend. There will be times during lowered immunity where it will not be possible to bring in outside food. But, while it was possible, I made sure to supplement the rather plain hospital fare with other tasty food. However, a lack of appetite can also be common during severe chemo treatments.

There were times when I would just sit in a chair in the room and read a book or the newspaper. Cathy might doze or sleep. There were even a couple of times when the nurses brought in a mattress for me to sleep in the room late into the night. I would be there if she woke up, we might chat for a while, and then repeat the cycle. I would disappear to have a coffee in the hospital café and watch the passing parade of patients and visitors.

There were times when Cathy needed to be angry, frustrated and quite overwhelmed with what was happening to her. Letting her express these feelings was vital. I was often amazed at her resilience and capacity to be so patient. But there were times when it all became too much. On one occasion the nurse could not find a vein to take blood, and I arrived to find her deeply distressed and saying through tears she could not take it anymore. I went to talk quietly to the nursing staff to understand what was happening and if this could be managed differently. This ultimately resolved itself, but it's important to recognize that being in hospital for a life-threatening illness is a very difficult experience, and just listening to Cathy vent (although I must add it was not often) was helpful.

You will need to censor yourself from time to time in order not to unduly worry your partner or friend. Let them verbalise and express their feelings. They don't need to censor what they say, even if it is upsetting for you. Let them be frightened, vulnerable, angry etc. On the other hand, you should not hide your feelings completely in this process. Acknowledge your feelings too. You are, after all, not a robot. But again, try not to unnecessarily burden them if you are struggling.

I thought Cathy was incredibly brave; dealing with it day to day. Facing the possibility she might die, managing her needle phobia, the endless side effects of the chemo, then ICU and the stem cell transplant. She was feeling so weak a lot of the time. It seemed to go on and on. I think her innate capacity to approach the long term by taking things day-by-day was crucial. That takes great patience in my view.

Being actively engaged with the hospital staff (nurses, doctors and other ancillary professionals) and her treatment was also imperative. The Alfred staff always amazed me with their commitment and care. I wanted to know as much as possible, and I was often there when the medical team arrived for the daily consultation. If you have the difficult experience of the Intensive Care Unit, engaging with the nurses in the room will be amazingly informative and helpful in understanding what is happening. A positive relationship with them helps you as well.

Balancing a full-time job, along with daily hospital visits, sometimes both in the morning before work and after work into the evening, can be quite challenging and tiring. I was deeply grateful that I had a couple of close friends who helped and supported me. Having them around gave me strength. As a principal carer, you need to be looked after too. If you find yourself alone in this role maybe seek support professionally from a healthcare worker, and don't ignore the signs of anxiety, stress and exhaustion. You are not going to be much help if you collapse under the pressure of maintaining your own life. Don't deny you have strong feelings too. You will probably be frightened and overwhelmed, and your significant other is not in a place to help and support you. Take care of yourself, and don't act like a super person with super powers. You need rest, good food and a way to manage your own anxiety and stress.

I was at work most of the time as usual – although I took occasional days off. Being at work was good in a way; I had things to do but at times it was tiring and mentally exhausting. But as time went on I developed a daily routine.

The routine helped me feel better, knowing what I had to do in advance. There seemed so much uncertainty about it all. At least I was organised and I had a timetable and tasks every day, so it was not all chaos.

The realisation that she might die was a huge moment and the thought that I might be left alone was shocking. This led to me looking at our relationship in a different light and reinforced how special I thought it was. I also said we needed to get married as soon as the treatment was over. We had been together for thirty-seven years and had often joked about not being ready. Getting married was a way of saying how much she meant to me, but also emphasising that she would get well and we would both be going on into the future.

Overall, we both ended up with a more focussed perspective on what was of consequence to us individually and together. It's a cliché, but life is short and there are a lot of distractions. We needed to focus on each other, the essential things and the special people around us.

ELEVEN

Things that pulled me through

Anyone dealing with cancer or come to think of it anyone dealing with any illness has to find strategies to make the experience more bearable. Obviously the approach taken will vary depending on personality and circumstance. When I was feeling nauseous after chemo or cracking up dealing with diabetes and injecting insulin my approach was to lie there and ride it out. Occasionally I felt so awful I wanted to give up and become unconscious. In this state no activity was enjoyable.

I made this list of the specific factors which contributed to my recovery. It is a surprisingly long inventory because it took a village, or in my case a small metropolis:

· My anonymous stem cell donor and every blood donor

· Accepting I was in for the long haul, with anxiety, and fatigue (not ordinary tiredness) my constant companions in the early days

· Attempting to live day to day, living with feelings of hope and gratitude mixed in with anger, despair and terror

- Not imposing positive thinking on myself
- Fred's love, patience and care
- The love and support of my family and friends
- The Alfred Hospital's exceptional medical care/ Medicare, our universal health insurance scheme
- Having the same medical professionals supervising my care from diagnosis onwards
- Following the treatment regime and learning to manage boredom and feeling sick
- Pharmacy medicines and plenty of them. Mixed in with vitamin supplements as required
- Learning to manage my fear of injections and hospital procedures. The gift of the Hickman and PICC lines and dialysis port
- Having a healthy, resilient body/the genetic lottery/good nutrition/exercise (I should have done extra workouts)
- Advocating for myself
- A creative life and an active imagination/a sense of humour/ curiosity
- Time at home to heal and rest without added stress but with the benefits of massages and sleep
- Coffee
- Hypnotherapy
- The healing power of music
- Reading.
- Researching and writing my various books
- Making time to travel and visit friends

· My garden – a pesticide free haven

· Gus the tabby cat.

The emerging writer

Slowly my energy levels improved. I could do more than lie about on the couch vegetating like a potato (no offence to potatoes).

I have always been someone who liked to create and keep busy; everything from sewing my own clothes to gardening to photography. Now I had developed a new skill. I love reading. And thanks to the cancer I now adore writing. I have the archives of Dorothy Armitage Rudder, a great aunt of Fred's, to thank for my new found occupation. Writing her biography, *Dainty Diva*, gave me the momentum and resolution to share my own story.

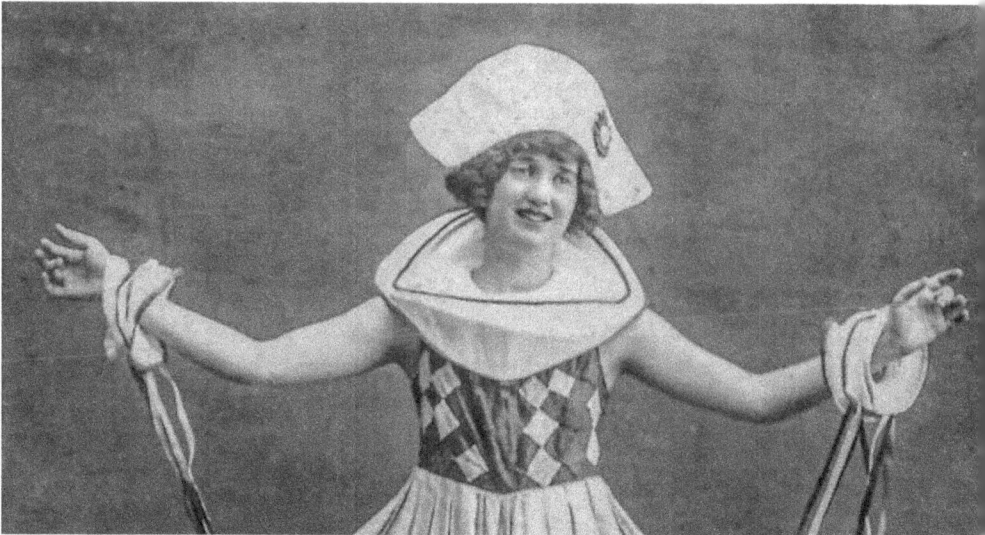

Dorothy Rudder, Sydney soprano and variety theatre artist. Photo by Gordon and Blees Calcutta 1919.

Years ago a special brown suitcase came into my life. Upon opening the suitcase my initial reaction was fascination mixed with an oddly non-defined feeling of melancholy. Someone's life was being laid bare. It sat there, a one of these days when I have more time project. Finally, owing to the little c, I could properly investigate the contents. A whole new world opened up, giving me the opportunity to navel gaze about something other than myself and the endless tedious emphasis on getting well.

I positioned the computer at the dining room table, sat facing out toward the garden and commenced organising the materials in date order. I took plenty of mini rests. I then typed up a selection of letters and her diary from her 1919 Far East theatrical tour and created performance and radio broadcast timelines. It was now time to trawl the internet. Exciting surprises were in store.

Dorothy was a beguiling, tenacious and feisty Australian woman. Hers is a poignant story where lost opportunities as well as successes played an integral part. She was compelled to perform no matter what life threw in her path, from the inherent insecurity of a stage career to a sensational divorce and the massive personal fallout from two world wars. I was intrigued.

The research would have been impossible without access to organisations such as the National Library of Australia which hosts Trove, a massive free archive of digitised resource material. Through Trove I discovered many mentions of Dorothy in contemporary newspapers. By lucky chance I discovered some copies of her letters on eBay UK and also obtained copies of her divorce papers which included the actual testimony of Dorothy and husband Len Smith in the NSW Supreme Court. It made for compelling reading! Early in the piece the project was assisted by a grant from the Royal Australian Historical Society. Being awarded this small grant gave me the impetus to keep researching. Someone else believed my explorations were worthwhile.

In Dorothy Rudder's suitcase was a document of particular interest for me; an expensively produced program for a cancer fundraiser. At the age of forty-three, after years of working in Australia in the opera chorus and on the concert platform, Dorothy decided to try her luck in England. London's New Scala Theatre was the venue for the Middlesex Hospital 43rd Annual Variety Concert on 23 November 1937 in aid of their cancer wing. The line-up of acts was notable, and apart from Dorothy included such entertainment luminaries of the time as Arthur Askey, George Formby (famous for his rendition of *When I'm cleaning windows*), acrobatic dancers Newman, Wheeler and Yvonne (check out their act on YouTube and be amazed), and renowned band leader Jack Hylton.

The Middlesex Hospital's Consulting Surgeon wrote a page on cancer treatment for the program which made me think about my own experience and current advances in cancer research. He thought the crab, the symbol of cancer, an inhuman creature with horrid eyes and remorseless claws, had not been killed but turned over on its back and its claws rendered harmless. There were no stem cells transplants in the 1930s. When I finished writing *Dainty Diva* I had a huge sense of accomplishment as I sent her story out for the world to read. (Details of where to find it are at the end of this book.)

Once my first book was completed I contemplated what to write about next. I know, I'll write the story of my cancer encounter. But first, an article based on some incredible stories of animals performing on the vaudeville stage in Australian and New Zealand that I came across while researching *Dainty Diva*. These acts often comprised dogs, cats, birds and monkeys. However, a virtual riot of unusual animals was also working hard for a crust including an anteater, although its act was probably a slow one. I had the thrill of seeing a lead article based on this research – 'Antipodean Animal Acts' – published in the National Library of Australia's online magazine *Unbound*, March 2019. I proudly gave a printed copy to Professor Curtis and Nurse Georgia because without their care this article would never have seen the light of day.

Writing my story

One unquestionably beautiful thing has come out of the cancer. Without my donor's precious, life-saving gift I wouldn't be writing this now.

Writing my story has led to a fundamental question. How did I manage to overcome Acute Myeloid Leukaemia and all the associated complications of treatment? As illustrated by the list of specific factors which led to my recovery, so many circumstances came into play which determined my prospects of survival. After chemotherapy, although technically in remission, I was not cancer free. However, the donor's precious, healthy new cells eliminated the faulty cells that my immune system was unable to mop up, turning my vague hopes of survival into reality.

I remind myself that the figures thrown about regarding survival rates are somewhat rubbery. They look at the average person and the figures can vary widely depending on the source. I am not necessarily 'average'; I don't think any blood cancer patient is average, from the genetic profile of their disease to their age, overall health or the way they cope with procedures or GVHD. I was reminded of this when undergoing chemo. Some patients in the ward did not experience any nausea. This made me so envious. Meanwhile, even though I had access to anti-nausea drugs, I vomited on and off for weeks. I also gagged when eating certain foods (the type of food rejected could vary from day to day), unpleasant smells, sights such as cat vomit or even when cleaning my teeth.

Travel – Europe by B&B

Travel has always been a predominant part of my life with Fred. We don't have children and have spent many a house deposit on exciting journeys to Europe, the United States, Canada, Asia and the one country we visited in Africa – Morocco. The bug started to bite again, made affordable by a small inheritance from my mother. In July 2013 we headed for Europe with a stopover in Singapore. It was only ten months after my stem cell procedure. My energy level was way lower than a so-called normal person's and I feared being so far away from The Alfred. What if I ended up in a hospital in Paris? Do the doctors there deal with AML in the same way? Can I explain my symptoms properly? Will my hospital bed have a view of the

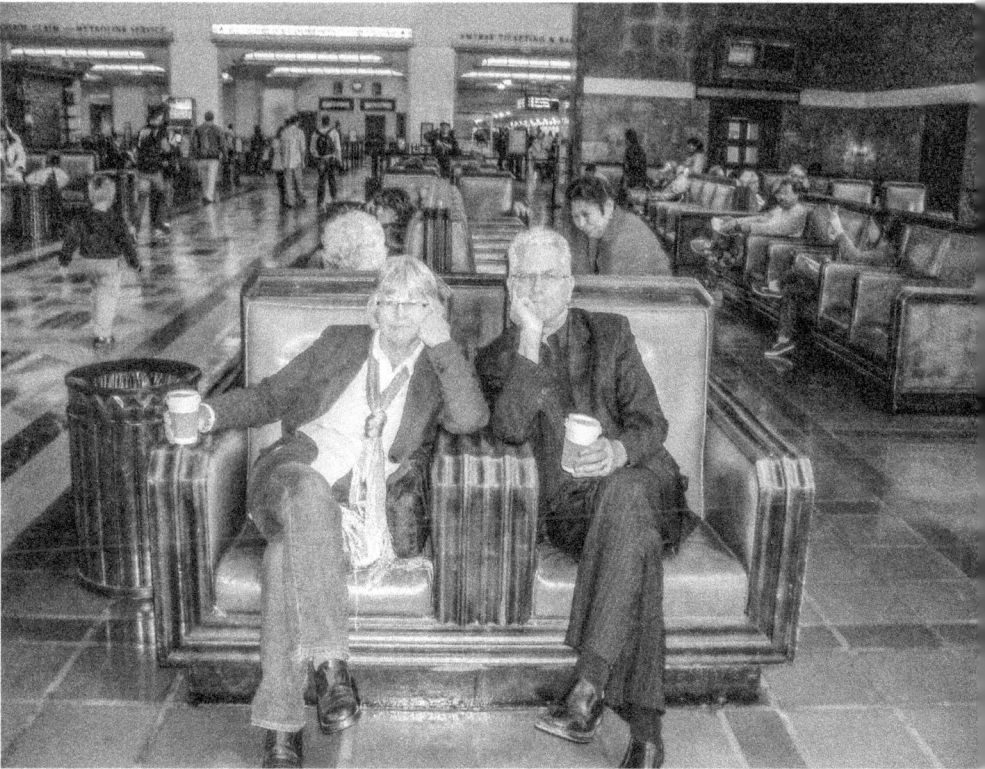

Union Station Los Angeles 2010.

Eiffel Tower? Then I thought – Of course they do. Of course I can. Fred could sure use a holiday too. Let's go for it.

Professor Curtis saw no problem with our travel plans. Although Lloyds of London refused to insure me because of the pre-existing cancer (I like to be rejected by the most prestigious companies), I took comfort in the fact that any bad symptoms would take time to develop. Time enough to get back home and crawl into my own hospital bed at The Alfred if I needed to.

Half the fun of travel is planning the itinerary and we decided to go the high-end B&B route. Amsterdam, Paris, Lille, Bologna, London and York were all memorable. We took the time to visit the Australian WWI Memorial at Villers-Bretonneux where, in July 1938, Dorothy Rudder was one of the 3,500 attendees at the memorial's inauguration as her brother was listed on the commemorative wall. The memorial is an austerely beautiful Art Deco style structure which overlooks a vast plain outside the town, standing on high ground above the Military Cemetery where Commonwealth servicemen who died on the surrounding battlefields during the First World War are buried. This was also the trip where we brought Mum's ashes home to her Dutch village.

Travel – Yosemite National Park

Putting fears of relapse to the back of our minds, and obtaining travel insurance with various exclusions, late in 2016 Fred and I visited Jim and Paulette in San Francisco.

Our trip to the Sierra Nevada included two special highlights. The Calaveras Big Trees State Park, home of the giant sequoias, is a short drive away from Jim and Paulette's cosy cabin. Many of the trees are huge; between 75 and 90 metres in height and 30 metres in circumference. The bark is thick and spongy, not hard like our eucalyptus trees. The feeling you get by standing underneath these magnificent trees is difficult to put into words. Looking up, all that can be seen is a massive canopy with tiny bits of sky poking through.

We spent a few days at Yosemite National Park in the depths of winter in 2016. Driving along the winding mountain roads was a memorable meditation tinged with sadness, as many large trees had died in the recent drought. Giant redwoods, boulders, smaller trees and tiny shrubs were blanketed with a thick white powdery coating of snow, like a vast, icy fairyland. Every now and again we saw a deer, still as a statue as it watched us drive by.

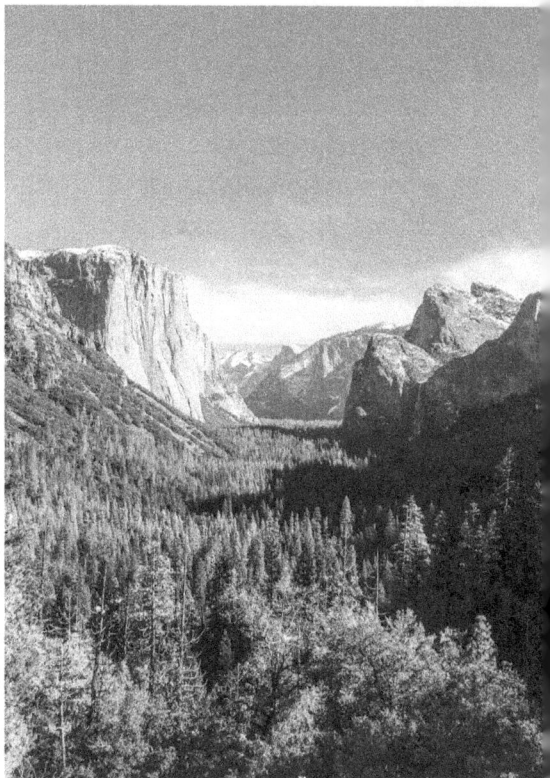

Yosemite National Park.

The importance of nature

Although I did not voice it to many people, during my hospitalisation two needs were often with me. I needed to go outside, and I needed my home in the country. When I was feeling strong enough, I could enjoy sitting in the wintery sun in the large park across the road from the hospital, wearing a hat and coat with a small block of chocolate stashed in my pocket. Since my recovery our country garden has provided this haven.

My garden is alive, a little bit wild and unpredictable and ever changing, in the Australian tradition, from lush lime green to dry and brown and back to green again. I have always been compelled to garden, but before I developed AML I did not see my garden as an essential ingredient in recovery from illness. Now I do. It strikes me that gardens are vitally important for our well-being because they involve all five senses. I can sit looking out at the trees and across the hillside; I can touch leaves and flowers, hear creatures communicating or foraging about for food, enjoy the fragrance of wet eucalyptus and savour the herbs for our meals.

I have a theory. The activities you love to do in childhood are an excellent indicator of the career path you should follow as an adult. I knitted dolls clothes from the age of three, made huts in the bush and created two editions of my own newspaper as a teenager. I wrote regular, if rudimentary, movie reviews in my diary along the lines of: The film was really good and I liked it a lot. As an adult I learned how to work complex paper patterns,

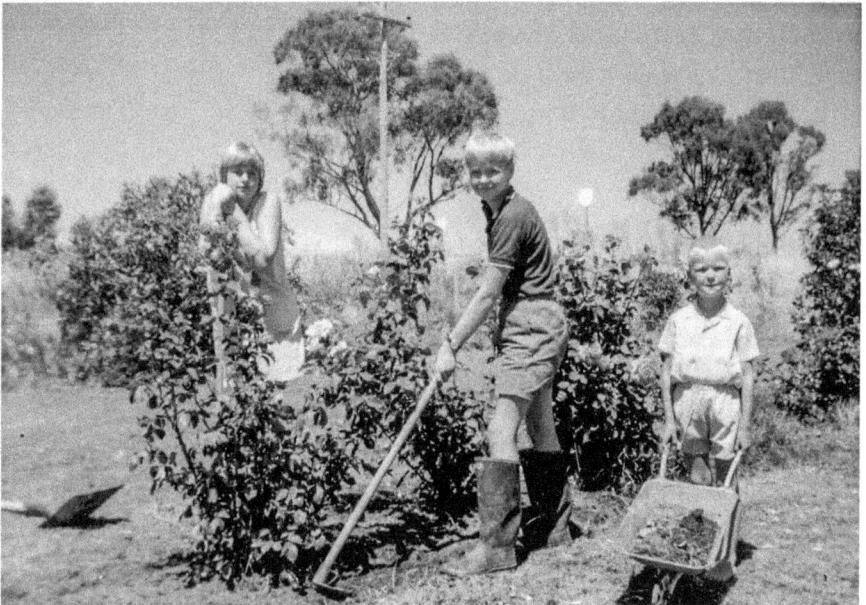

The reluctant gardeners.

mould the fabric and create my own clothes. I worked front of house and as a cinema publicist. At age eleven I cultivated a violet plant and carefully recorded the emergence of every flower into an exercise book. As you can imagine that soon palled but a love of plants never faded.

After gardening in a small, flat suburban plot with the neighbours only metres away, the half-hectare hillside property we bought fifteen years ago presented a huge challenge both for its size and topography. The soil is ancient granitic sand weathered away over the millennia. A short drive in any direction from our town offers dramatic vistas of enormous granite boulders, some balancing on tip-toes on other rocks. It's strange but I never used to think about the traditional Taungurung people, consisting of nine clans, whose land this is and who lived and cared for this special place long, long before Fred and I came here.

Now I imagine the ancestors of our district's clan, the Nira Balug or Cave People, walk across the heavily-treed landscape and head for the creek at the bottom of the hill. As they make the best use of their resource-rich environment they catch fish, collect berries, make shelters, baskets and nets for harvesting fat, brown Bogong Moths, along with spears and boomerangs for hunting animals such as kangaroos, wombats, koalas and emus. The landscape is no longer heavily-treed and there are no koalas or emus here now – I haven't seen a possum for years. However, large mobs of kangaroos regularly visit our garden, especially in summer for an early evening drink out of the bird baths and to neatly trim the tops from the grasses and shrubs I have planted.

Our house is a wooden Californian Bungalow which was sliced in half, put onto trucks and relocated from suburban Melbourne. The previous owners covered the outer walls in brick and made improvements which provided the foundation for an organic, predominantly native garden. I aimed for a parklike effect; a strolling space with mulched paths and beds.

Rejuvenation was the name of this game.

While I worked with my friend Damian to make new paths, reshape garden beds and plant gum trees, shrubs and vegetables, Fred cooked up a storm in the kitchen, calling out to us.

'Lunch is ready. Let's eat on the front veranda.'

'What are we eating today? Spaghetti with asparagus and parmesan cheese? Vegetable lasagne? Or grilled sardines with tomatoes from the vegetable patch? What about some peaches from the orchard for dessert?'

My culinary and horticultural life was, and is, good.

When I first came out of hospital I found it difficult to garden. My energy was depleted and my balance was not great. This made it hard to dig, prune and mulch. Being faced with my own mortality had made me overly fearful. Possible dangers in the garden loomed ridiculously large in my thoughts, especially a brown snake biting me (well, they are Australia's most venomous snake and more than a few happen to call my garden home) or a kangaroo kickboxing me in the stomach. Going forth regularly between city and country did not help either because gardening requires continuity.

Slowly I regained my energy and began to reclaim the space.

My garden has taught me patience. Regular mulching, together with extensive tree planting, has created a much more fertile, friable soil and that has taken time. Many species of birds, bees, snakes, lizards, the odd echidna and emu, frogs, butterflies and many other insects have made the garden their home or come around for a seasonal visit, providing continuous opportunities to observe nature close up. I'm finding birds in particular wonderful to watch. Our baby magpies squawk at their parents with demands to be fed, technicolour parrots cavort in the birdbaths, bossy cockatoos flick their yellow crests, letting the rosellas know they were there first and honey eaters plunge their beaks deep into brush-like Grevillea flowers. I look up as a wedge tailed eagle soars nonchalantly above.

It is now the place to sniff the heady scent of the roses and lilacs, after checking for bees and other little creatures which might be foraging inside. Time to heal, build up my vitamin D levels, read a book, take a stroll with Fred or enjoy a glass of prosecco or chardonnay with friends and watch the way the shadows fall as the sun goes down. Or in one memorable incident, watch a large brown snake pursue a blue tongue lizard across the vegetable patch and slowly but surely swallow it whole, right below the back veranda. I was so engrossed in what I saw I forgot to photograph it for Facebook.

A new mindset

Looking at the big picture, after going through cancer (or should I say cancer going through me) my worries about the future of our planet have grown exponentially. Global deforestation, climate change, the continual threat of bushfires, heatwaves and storms, air pollution from burning fossil fuels, misuse of precious resources, the privatisation of natural monopolies, the mistreatment of animals, the scourge of plastic waste and continual economic growth as the only indicator of prosperity – it's death by a million cuts. A huge change of mindset is required and there are some heartening signs this is happening. I choose to make a small contribution by planting a large variety of native trees and shrubs. And by embracing the vision of naturalists such as David Attenborough and not those who greet the melting of polar ice sheets and shrinking glaciers as a fabulous mining opportunity.

Where's the bill?

Not having to be unduly concerned with the cost of my treatment is a huge benefit of living in Australia. Blood cancer is a costly affair for our public health system and yet treatment is made available to anyone who needs it for free or low cost. The total cost of treating and caring for all blood cancer patients in 2019 was a total of $3.4 billion over their lives and is expected to rise to over $10.9 billion in 2035.

Since my recovery a thought sometimes occurs when crossing a busy road. I have to be extra careful because, if a vehicle or bike collects me, all the money and effort spent on my survival would be wasted. I have read and been given figures from $334,000 to $1.5 million per patient. Although I have no exact figure for the cost of my medical treatment Professor Curtis tells me it was around $500,000. I underwent five bone marrow biopsies ($2,500 a procedure), had two Hickmans, two PICC lines and one dialysis line inserted, had endless blood tests, dialysis, infusions of plasma, magnesium, red blood cells and hydrating fluids and spent twenty-four days in ICU at $10,000 a day. My allogenic (donor) stem cell transplant cost around $125,000. And my treatment is still ongoing.

Add to this the cost of chemotherapy drugs, immunosuppressant drugs, tranquilisers, insulin, sterile dressings, syringes, swabs, diagnostic equipment, dialysis machines etc.

Although the treatment is free in public hospitals, and I am most thankful for that, cancer can still leave the patient with large out of pocket expenses and loss of income. AML took away future years of employment (I estimate lost salary at over $500,000) leaving me dependent on Fred's salary. Thank goodness he had secure employment although keeping on working was also a pressure for him. Spare a thought for families, especially those with young children, when the only wage earner is diagnosed with cancer. That is a frightening situation, both emotionally and economically. The Leukaemia Foundation reported how in 2018 only 14% of people living with blood cancer were able to continue working as they had before. I'm surprised it is that many. The cost of transport and accommodation for patients needing to travel long distances to treatment centres can also present big financial challenges.

My personal expenses included my two GPs, one in the country and another in the city (the first bulk billed, the other did not); hospital car parking and public transport, approximately $2,500 over six years (parking currently costs a maximum rate of $28 or $10 concession per day at The Alfred), TV and internet in the ward, purchases at The Alfred's newsagents/post office, Alf's café and the chemist for drugs.

The hospital covers the cost of drugs while in the ward but once you leave, you pay. Not to forget my sessions with a hypnotherapist, part of which was claimable on Medicare. I estimated spending around $160 monthly on drugs at The Alfred's outpatients' pharmacy (which processes prescriptions generated by Alfred Health doctors and specialists) and regular chemists until I went on the Aged Pension. I now pay only $6.60 a prescription. Fortunately, almost all of these drugs are listed on the Pharmaceutical Benefits Scheme (PBS). It is no secret drugs are big business. The cost of the PBS to the Australian Government was $12.6 billion in the 2019-2020 financial year, almost double the $6.7 billion cost in 2007.

Be Patient

I've lost count of the number of hospital days and outpatient visits I have made. Alfred Health staff saw 239,033 patients at their Outpatients Departments in 2019-20. I accounted for a few of those visits with most of those happening on weekday mornings or afternoons.

From my experience as a public patient in a public hospital, waiting is normal. It is not called the waiting room for nothing, but the fact this is available to Australians for free makes the waiting worth it. Be prepared and bring along a good book (not *War and Peace*, it's a bit long) your mobile phone, a magazine or Sudoku. Even a game of chess could work, as long as you don't spend too much time staring at the board. You may be there for an hour or two. I don't mind; I'm pleased to be looked after by so many expert doctors and I have the flexibility to plan my appointments. It may be a different story for those with a job to go to or children to collect from school. Blood tests are often required and wait times can vary. There are no appointments at The Alfred's Blood Collection Centre; it is first come first served. After presenting my pathology slip from the doctor plus my Medicare card, I can occasionally go straight in. At other times the waiting area is packed.

Who's involved?

It is the medical personnel who are the centre of my clinical care and I will always be grateful to them. I made a list of everyone who looked after me. Numero uno is the Professor and the nurses, in particular specialist transplant nurses Georgia, Daniela and Bianca who have overseen my care to this day; teams of specialist doctors – ICU, haematologists, Late Effects Clinic, heart, lung and osteoporosis specialists, researchers; the teams who insert catheters such as Hickmans and PICCs, the nurses in the wards and ICU – all staffed day and night and every public holiday; staff in the Emergency Department; the rehabilitation hospital workers; the phlebotomists doing innumerable blood tests and the pathology team who analyse the results; the radiographers and doctors involved with mammograms, dialysis, heart and lung scans and bone density tests; the surgeons undertaking colonoscopies, the therapists; endocrinologists and diabetes educators; the receptionists; the cleaners; the orderlies, the social workers; the catering staff; the laundry workers; the hospital dentist; the staff at The Alfred's outpatient pharmacy; the X-ray team for oral and chest X-rays; the ambulance service; the Blood Bank; my GP and the staff at the local clinic; the podiatrist; the optometrist; the heart specialists; the skin specialists and Nexus Primary Health staff. I hope I haven't forgotten anybody. I can't add the florist because flowers could not be brought into the ward and visiting priests and volunteers are not paid for under the hospital system.

It struck me that medical care can be looked at from another side of the ledger too, as a profitable business. My ongoing encounter with AML has become a substantial generator of income in the community, providing work for many people at The Alfred and beyond, with most of the costs ultimately covered by the taxpayer.

Although it is mutually beneficial, I won't go as far as to say it is 'win win' because as you know, I am trying to live my best cliché-free life. Let's just say we're happily in a long-term symbiotic relationship.

Helping with Research

In addition to treating patients The Alfred is a major teaching and research institution. I was impressed by the nearly 180 research posters displayed on the ground floor of the hospital in June 2018 covering topics such as infectious diseases, cardiovascular disease, mental health, nursing and allied health. Being able to give something back, to assist in this critical research, was imperative to me, so to support The Alfred's work I participated in the following research projects. I haven't been involved in any clinical trials of new drugs; only 20% of blood cancer patients participate in these.

· Collection and Storage of Blood Samples at the ABMDR Tissue Repository 2012. I donated quite a few vials of blood for this project.

· Exploring the Factors predicting Psychological Distress and Health-related Quality of Life in Haematopoietic Stem Cell Transplant May 2012

- Filter Life in Renal Replacement Therapy 2012. This was the project Fred signed up for on my behalf in ICU.
- Nutrition in Blood Cancer Survivors study 2017
- Cancer Survivors and Support Persons' Preferences for Care: A Discrete Choice Experiment. February 2017

Furthermore, the important research carried out by hospitals such as The Alfred always requires substantial injections of funding. Fred and I have left a bequest in our wills and I would encourage others to also support this type of vital work.

TWELVE

Who am I now?

Feeling sorry for myself

Seven years after the diagnosis I turned into a big sook and felt guilty about it. I found all the visits to the specialists hard to take, even though I was thankful for their care. Being a good patient and doing all the right things in order to keep alive still felt like hard work. I was under obligation to ensure I took the prescribed tablets, did the insulin injections, turned up to appointments on the right day and on time, made sure I had a blood test and many other tests as well. I was, and still am, in an important relationship not just with Professor Curtis but with The Alfred Hospital and the entire medical system. If I messed up and stop playing by the rules I would be kicked out of the club. When would it end?

Although I did admit it evolved into a positive learning experience to an extent, I became fed up with having to deal with a new symptom every few months, year after year. My apple a day did not keep the doctors away but I couldn't go around kicking and punching doctors and nurses like I did at three when they took my tonsils out. I grizzled to the Professor on my next visit. I asked him when I could get off the steroids when I knew they were needed to counteract the GVHD. I now sounded like a boring old record, the same request played over and over.

I contemplated longer term therapy but didn't do anything about it. I should have had further psychiatric assistance in the first two years after diagnosis. I was my own worst enemy in this regard; coping not only with debilitating symptoms pre-diagnosis, the chemo and the three weeks of ICU but also the death of my mother, Fred's risky heart bypass, moving house twice, the GVHD and the side effects of the drugs to counteract it, needle phobia and not being able to work. I took the stoic approach, thinking I would use my own inner resources to deal with whatever was thrown at me. And now my resources were feeling very threadbare.

I wanted to go back to normal; how I lived my life before this whole AML thing kicked me up the bum. Well, I told myself that was never going to happen. I reminded myself my quality of life was still high. I continued to garden, drive a car and enjoy Fred's delicious cooking. I wrote and read to my heart's content, listened to music, saw movies with friends, laughed out loud and followed a footy team (Geelong Cats of course). I regularly travelled about the place. And although Mum was no longer with us and I still missed her, I could now cook a fillet steak in butter almost as well as she did. I was still doing all the things I said I would miss when originally diagnosed, when I faced death. Come on Cathy. Stop whining. Snap out of it.

Was my body dealing with some GVHD, supressed injecting fears, too many months on the Prednisolone or had I caught a bug? What was going on in that body of mine that I used to take for granted? Time to retreat to the protection of my bed once more, get on the horse again and ride it out. Time to be immobile, go flat, be like a pupa in its cocoon. Time to retreat sideways back into the crab cave. Because as a cancer patient you have to be flexible enough to make the same manoeuvres as a crab, mentally at least. And hang on for dear life with your claws.

What if this sick feeling did not retreat? What if I had to keep taking Prednisolone for life? How would I manage the daily insulin injections this third time round? I would have to find out.

After three days of wallowing, part of my usual pattern of coping, I metamorphosed. I felt much better and more optimistic. To some extent.

I caught up with Nurse Georgia in May 2019 and she checked my vital signs. Although my blood pressure was up, I didn't stress as this happened occasionally. I didn't want to start on blood pressure tablets though. My pulse was thankfully back to normal and my temperature and oxygenation levels were good. The first thing Professor Curtis said when he saw me was – 'you're looking good.' Ditto, I thought. He looked at rows and rows of numbers on his computer screen. For the first two years after the transplant, engrafting and blood level numbers were of prime importance because transplants do not always work. I now took it for granted that my blood readings would be normal and worried about my kidneys and liver instead (and if they were OK, I would find another body part to be fearful about). The Professor analysed the numbers and was pleased because these organs had markedly improved from the February readings. He wrote down the words – seven years post-transplant, in the clinical notes box of the blood test request form I needed for my next appointment. As we wrapped up the consultation the Professor declared, 'Seven years! All things considered you have done really well. You are well and truly cured of leukaemia and there is very little chance of it coming back.' Elephant stamp, go straight to the top of the class.

Without any proof I had a feeling my donor's cells were slowly giving up their takeover attempts, although I accepted I would have more bouts of GVHD and might be on immunosuppressant drugs for the rest of my life. But to be honest a small part of me wanted to stop taking all these tablets, eat bucket loads of sugary products, overdo the alcoholic drinks and sit in the sun all day. I lie. A *large* part of me sometimes wanted to chuck the tablets right out the bathroom window.

July 2019

Kidneys looking good, liver alright, red cell levels fine, white cells slightly elevated but Professor Curtis thought this was due to the Prednisolone. The pred. and insulin levels were now lowered. I would be off them soon.

2020, Coronavirus pandemic strikes

The world-wide spread of Covid-19 led to restrictions that particularly affected my relatives in The Netherlands but did not alter our lives to the same extent. We coped with the lockdowns because we were retired, didn't run a business and lived in the countryside which suffered fewer restrictions than the cities. That said, we were still in a higher risk category because of our age and health issues and had to be careful. Masking and vaccinations were non-negotiable.

The hermit crab lifestyle quite suited me. However, every time I turned on the TV an image popped up of someone's unsheathed arm being jabbed with a needle (and I heard the phrase, new normal, get another test run). Although only momentarily disturbed, I wondered how others with medical phobias coped. I did enjoy the close up illustrations of the virus with its pretty sucker-like florets popping out all over the surface. It reminded me of a weird spaceship or a stunning flower you might expect to find emerging from a succulent.

We managed to escape to northern NSW for Christmas and just made it back home before a full lockdown was declared. The ten days of required isolation were easy, the free Covid test not so much. I let out a high-pitched squeal when the long, Q-tip like swab unexpectedly went all the way up my nose.

A plethora of doctors' appointments
and some big news

Proudly taking an active role in my own care, in October 2020 I emailed Professor Curtis voicing some concerns.

I am worried about long term effects of tacrolimus on my compromised kidneys but also know I have to keep the GVHD under control. But how much of an issue is GVHD for me after eight years? I guess the next blood test will tell us more.

In May 2021 I received big news; news I had wanted to hear for such a long time. Professor Curtis declared me GVHD free. After nearly nine years of carefully managing side effects this was a special moment. Farewell and goodbye to the daily popping of immunosuppressant drugs. No more worrying about the donor cells tussling for supremacy with my cells. A truce had been declared.

In a victory of sorts I now saw the Professor every six months rather than every two or three months. However new health issues crept sneakily into the equation due to the inevitability of maturing, of getting older. Nature was taking its course and my body, like that of many of my friends, was slowly wearing out. Although his elegant tabby and white fur coat covered up any protruding bones or sagging skin and he was still quite fit, even Gus the cat was now classified as geriatric at sixteen years.

An astonishing number of tests instigated by my GP, The Alfred and on occasion courageously even booked by me, revealed mixed results. If I was a car, this would be called a major service and repair job. I wished I could trade in my body for a new and younger model. Each time I awaited the test results I quaked in my boots and couldn't sleep the night before. After nine years the theme, and my response to it, was becoming somewhat repetitive, even boring. Once more I asked – What next? I thought I might have finally reached the end of the line and once more I gave thanks to our medical system for helping to keep me alive.

First I underwent investigations on my heart. At the podiatrist of all places a monitoring clip placed onto my big toe registered some heart palpitations! And yes, I could feel my heart skipping a beat when I lay in bed. I wore a holter monitor to track the heart's rhythm for twenty-four hours. Yes, the beat was irregular and I thought stress seemed to be a factor. A follow-up echocardiogram showed the heart was normal but the palpitations needed to be dealt with. My GP put me on beta-blockers which work by preventing the stress-related hormone adrenaline from making my heart pump quicker or with more force. This lowered my blood pressure and reduced the palpitations markedly. He still wanted the irregular heartbeats to be checked out to cover all the bases so I saw a specialist. The next appointment required a stress test which involved a treadmill, the onset of shortness of breath due to my compromised lungs and another echocardiogram. The image of my heart on the screen came out fuzzy. When the doctor told me I needed to go to another clinic where the treadmill test would be repeated using a special injection of a tiny amount of radioactive tracing material you could imagine my thoughts. What the hell? Not more tests! When I returned home I reminded myself that my father had died of heart disease and Fred had a hard time with his heart issues. I was fortunate to be offered these tests and if they found anything amiss it was advantageous to catch it early.

I was impressed with the hospital gown offered at the second clinic. Soft blue cotton, nice to wear and not disposed of after one short single use, in contrast to other medical clinics. I did not impress myself by feeling strange in the head and nearly fainting on the treadmill. A few days later my GP gave me the best news. He confirmed my heart worked just fine, quite tip top in fact. What a relief! It was news I desperately needed. I couldn't wait to tell Fred who had patiently listened to me predict my potential demise, this time via ectopic heartbeats and heart failure.

Next up, another DEXA scan of the hip and spine revealed that osteopenia had turned into osteoporosis. The bones had become more brittle due to a reduction in their density. Blame menopause and prolonged steroid use for this one. Weight bearing exercises and an intravenous infusion of zoledronic acid, a drug which slows down bone turnover, allowing the cells time to rebuild some new bone, were in my immediate future. Then, an ultrasound to investigate elevated liver enzymes revealed a fatty liver and pancreas. I was still diabetic but thankfully it was now controlled by a drug in tablet form, not insulin. Losing some weight became a priority. On the positive side of the ledger, no problems were revealed after a bladder ultrasound, skin check or eye examination.

Next I had four small fillings on my front teeth, all in one go, and made a wonderful and surprising discovery. Since my last, painful injection into the gums decades ago, the technology had moved on. The dentist rubbed in a numbing potion before he injected and I didn't feel a thing until I received the bill.

I haven't yet mentioned the biggest procedure – I conscientiously sent off my bowel cancer test sample in the mail confidently expecting no issues but the result showed a little blood. Taking up my default position I assumed the worst but reminded myself colon cancer had an excellent survival rate when caught early. A colonoscopy followed at the local hospital where a single group of non-cancerous polyps were removed and minor diverticulitis found. The concoction taken earlier to clear the bowels, for some obscure reason labelled tropical fruit, made me vomit – violently and inelegantly. Fortunately this did not affect the outcome. And, I'm pleased to say I handled the procedure well. A nurse gently held my hand and rubbed my back as I went under which I found quite comforting.

Mother Nature's lessons

June 2021. Fred and I congratulated ourselves on getting the garden into brilliant order after sixteen years. But not so fast; nature is running this show; you only think you are. A few days later a massive storm hit the district, unlike any we had previously experienced. The wind, which registered an average of 110 kilometres an hour, intermittently roared through like a freight train. Stop, start, stop, start – howling and swirling for sixteen long hours. The power failed and I lay in bed holding my breath in trepidation, just like I did in hospital. Sleep was impossible. A walk around the garden the next morning exposed a scene of some devastation with two gum trees ripped straight from the ground roots and all, large tree branches strewn everywhere and solid concrete tiles blown right off the roof. A tidy up revealed most of the plants survived the onslaught and we now had a good supply of firewood for next year. It took a few days for the feeling of uneasiness to subside.

After the storm it struck me that although many gardeners valiantly attempt to keep garden beds and lawns tidy and love to plant out box hedges in neat soldierly rows, nature is inherently messy. This seeming chaos is essential for both plants and animals. It allows tree hollows to form and creates debris which provides habitat and sustenance for the next generation of growth. And talking about garden debris, while raking leaves near the shed I noticed the weight under the rake suddenly increase and discovered a 30cm long blue tongue lizard all caught up in the teeth. I gently touched its back. It puffed up, flattened out and looked dead for some time. Fortunately no harm was done. It likes to sunbake and I like to sneak up on it and see how long it takes for my new reptilian friend to scurry off when it senses I'm around.

A birthday to celebrate

I'm slowly coming to terms with turning seventy next year.

Ideas for celebrating seven decades on the planet, the ten precious years since diagnosis and the ten years since I married Fred, swirl around. I said adios and finito to my life after the doctor declared I had leukaemia. But I was premature in my conclusion. I was given a second and then a third chance. I'm still here. Despite everything that's happened I live normally and generally have good energy levels. I'm grateful for what I have. Even though I'm more mature I still have a future. I still have my dreams.

A change in awareness

Before the AML experience I used to walk through life to some degree in black and white, especially when out and about in the street. I did not always make connections between events. I was often oblivious to the actions of strangers; not always fully aware of my surroundings. Unless I needed to be, for example when running my horticulture business where attention to detail counted, I was often absorbed in my own thoughts – Cha Cha-ing my way through life.

This has changed since the little c, especially on public transport and when shopping. I now have more awareness, sometimes too much. I notice subtle colours; the way light falls on buildings. I'm more curious in general. I look into people's faces and reflect on the vibe they are putting out. Are they happy or miserable? Boring and loud conversations on mobiles make me want to join in to annoy the speaker. I notice how some pedestrians walk around as if they are the only ones in the street and contemplate how easy it would be to steal their handbags or wallets. I also notice the friendliness of workers who serve in my local shops and try to return the sentiment.

The Topic of Cancer – Who did I tell?

As previously touched upon, I never kept the cancer a secret from family and friends but after I came out of hospital I did not broadcast it either. In 2015 I decided to join the big wide world of social media, in other words Facebook. It was marvellous keeping up with my circle and learning many new things about their interests and opinions. My niece Danielle married Ben and we later welcomed Christopher into our lives; my brother Peter remarried and other family members including niece Stephanie were finding success in their jobs both at home and overseas. Some had travelled to Iran, Morocco, Europe, Japan, China and Vietnam and I vicariously shared in their adventures; friends celebrated special milestones, made stunning art or completed a pentathlon. I created a page for myself and another for my book *Dainty Diva*. I still wasn't interested in sharing my cancer story with the wider world, or overcooking tales of my ongoing roller coaster ride to my friends. I preferred to go under the radar while I recovered. By 2018 it felt right to invade my own privacy and commence writing this book. What did I have to lose, I thought? Maybe my tale could aid others dealing with blood cancer, either as patients, caregivers or friends.

A new attitude

I do have a changed attitude to life now, in part because I have been forced to adjust. It is possible to lose your health and find it again too, in a new way. It took some time to rediscover because I have to accept my physical limitations. I am more curious and engaged politically. I appreciate my loved ones more, have given up the full-time job search struggle and reinvented myself as an author. I have more time to enjoy and appreciate the large and small pleasures of life but this would have happened anyway as I reached retirement age.

I think about entropy – the inevitable decline from order into disorder – when I see my messy kitchen sink or a garden bed full of weeds once again. Maybe cancer is a kind of entropy too.

I have learned that the saying, if you lose your health you lose everything, needs a caveat. Although illness is unwelcome, I am not a total loser just because I became ill. Although living day to day can be difficult when feeling sick, I can still live a satisfying life and be a legend in my own lunchtime.

I still sweat the small stuff, although the line between small and big stuff is blurry nowadays. Take for instance the myriad requests for online reviews or surveys of products and services. It's technically small beer; no big deal. But, I don't want to spend time and energy reviewing every restaurant, hotel or product I have ever paid for. Life's too short, as my mum used to say. And when I have made an effort and forwarded negative feedback it is generally ignored. What if hospitals asked for a hotel-style review after each visit? I imagined what I'd say:

Bed quite a small single; shared a room with a complete stranger who didn't look very well. Sitting area windowless, magazines out of date, artwork a generic cityscape. Ordered a strong gin and tonic with dinner but it did not arrive. Enjoyed the vegemite on white bread, roast chicken and custard with cream. Life-saving platelet transfusion and a selection of tablets nicely delivered by friendly staff. However, I was woken up in the middle of the night for obs. and reception staff did not complete paperwork for check out until another five days had elapsed.

I received a valuable lesson about sweating the small stuff while on a Sunday drive in 2005. Fred and I decided to check out an antique shop in a nearby country town. The large Victorian-style house had a classic layout of long central corridor with spacious rooms leading off. Another couple stood at the counter, handing over $600 cash for an ornate Venetian mirror. The shop owner had placed the mirror in the doorway of the front room, ready for collection. It was balanced at a precarious angle on the corner of the door trim, not flat against the wall. You can imagine what was coming next. I saw the mirror as I walked out of the room but my overcoat just caught the edge. Result – a hundred pieces of lovely etched glass shattered as they hit the floor, transforming instantly into not-so-lovely pieces of useless junk. Everyone was mortified; however no glue in the world was going to put that mirror together again. I apologised profusely to the buyers and to the proprietor and offered to compensate for the loss. I will never forget her reply. 'You don't need to pay. I have just survived breast cancer. Something like this is just not significant compared to that.' Seven years later, following my encounter with the tenacious claws of the crab, I had my own opportunity to contemplate the true meaning of these words and how your perspective on what's important in life can alter after surviving a major illness.

We all experience difficult times of one sort or another. Priorities change and resilience and perseverance are sorely tested. I learned this a few years before the AML when a theatrical venture of Fred's went belly-up. We had to sell our lovely Californian Bungalow in Melbourne along with its lush garden which I had filled with rare plants. That was a huge financial and emotional loss; a challenging time for both of us. The only option was to start again and this led to our initial move to the country. I still ran my gardening business for a while but the commuting became too much and I ended up selling it. We managed to reinvent our lives by finding work locally and eventually buying another property. Over time a stressful experience, which I dealt with because I had to, unexpectedly evolved into a rewarding experience. In a strange way it made dealing with my illness a little easier.

Change is inevitable of course. I think it gives life its piquancy.

I have always loved making a nest, a safe haven, but since my illness this has become even more important. Out of curiosity I did a count of the number of homes I have lived in to date. They numbered twenty-six, including four in the last few years. I lived in nine houses before I left for university and attended six different schools. It all feels random and unpredictable.

I discovered that the experience of cancer is very different from what I thought it would be. Have you seen images of Niagara Falls? Do you recall Marilyn Monroe running around looking gorgeous in a yellow raincoat in the movie *Niagara*? Or viewed newsreel footage of punters hurtling over the falls in a barrel (good times

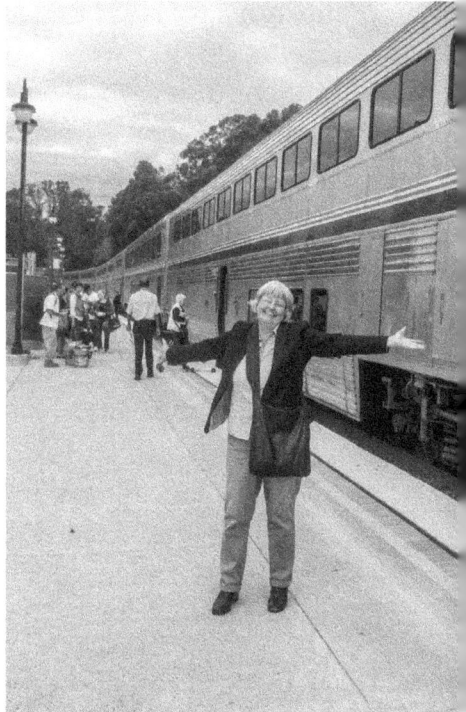

Happy en route from Los Angeles to San Francisco January 2015.

for all those who live to tell the tale) or crossing over the fast-flowing rapids by tightrope? Until I visited and donned a yellow raincoat myself, I always pictured this tourist attraction to be in the middle of nowhere, a wild and powerful place with no buildings in sight to mar the atmosphere. I discovered this perception was wrong. Especially when I found myself right near duty free shops, chocolate shops, adult stores and factory outlets, not to forget the odd casino or two.

Cancer is like that. I had fantasised about visiting the dreaded cancer place and how I would respond. The actual ordeal was nothing like I imagined. Given my childhood encounters with the world of medicine I was never going to be sanguine about it. I never thought hospitals could be a place of comfort and even amusement. Or that I would be able to roll up my sleeve and stoically accept a blood test, the insertion of an IV line or a flu or Covid vaccination. I never thought I would nearly die and live to tell about it or understand that cancer treatments can be a normal everyday part of life.

Cancer is not for sissies, milquetoasts, cowards or weaklings like me. Nevertheless, when cancer drops in for a visit there is no other choice. You have to confront it. You have to manage it. Dealing with cancer treatments is like running a one-person marathon. (I have read that some people don't like cancer being described as a marathon but I'm ok with it.) Your team and onlookers are cheering you on from the sidelines; you feel dehydrated and depleted; exhaustion kicks in; your team gives you a luridly coloured energy drink; you hit the wall then somehow your skinny body manages to keep on going; you fall over and pick yourself up again. The finish line is either the possibility of a cure or alternatively waking up under a cypress tree.

If I had my time again, knowing what I do now, would I still have chosen the stem cell transplant? Absolutely. All the signs were there that chemotherapy by itself was a temporary fix for the AML. The transplant was my only chance at a longer life. I am so fortunate to have been offered this option. Although medical issues have been my constant companion, I have managed, with support, to live an active and satisfying life and even travelled overseas four times. It is much harder to accept death now although I am more accepting of the possibility. However I don't want to contemplate any other cells mutating in my body.

My existence on this planet does feel that little bit sweeter. Like the gangster Johnny Rocco in the film *Key Largo* I want more. And like Rocco I will never have enough, time that is. Although I have been given an extra nine years so far, I still need more years. I have more people to play with, problems to solve, a few causes to grapple with. I am satisfied with what

I have materially. I don't need a bigger house, better food, or a brand new wardrobe of designer clothes. But I do need time to write more books. Three more are planned and I want to stay healthy and resilient for that. And I want to continue making sense of what happened to me, even if it is distressing.

> *To be resilient you need to be strong. You need a positive attitude and the ability to keep going when you encounter small setbacks. You need to be able to adapt well to change.*
>
> *You must accept reality (in my case stuck in Hospital longer than I would think is necessary).*
>
> *You need a deep belief in the outcome and have to back this up with strong values.*
>
> *You need to be able to improvise.*
>
> – Geoff Hamilton

Am I brave?

Although others, including Fred, have described me as brave, I often felt anything but brave. I do admit to reserves of resilience and courage. I have the ability to recover after experiencing stress, yet for me cancer was often an endurance test; a little visit to the darker side of life. My attitude during treatment could be hopeful, optimistic and accepting, at other times negative or irate. Sometimes I was in wait and see mode or in a neutral state. I did not pretend to be strong to stop others from worrying. Sometimes I was deeply depressed, feeling vulnerable, wallowing in the mire or ready to give up. Or pragmatic, just like my parents could be. Sometimes lateral thinking and daydreaming came to my rescue. The bottom line was I wanted to live so put up with whatever procedures came next. I jumped on the cancer bike and tried to stay on and keep peddling. Apart from occasionally visualising the cancer cells being knocked off deep inside my body by a dishwashing product shaped like a diamond, like I saw in a TV ad, or chomped by giant Pac-Men, I did not come equipped for battle because I did not have the energy or inclination to fight. I had no real expectation of being cured. If the dice rolled the right way and it wasn't loaded I might survive, if it came up cats' eyes it was goodbye world.

I took the chemotherapy treatments and waited (and waited) to see how they turned out. It was all about biology, my body's response and the change in the numbers. The blood readings were up or they were down, and up or down could both be good signs, depending on the aim of the treatment.

My AML was not a punishment, or an enemy to be hated. I did not cause my own cancer through having a devitalised mind. I did not need it, either consciously or subconsciously. In one swift pincer movement my body made some spare, but totally useless, chromosomes, a fiendishly clever but potentially deadly move for their host. Nobody really knows why this happened. I suspect it could be environmental damage and my genetic inheritance, combined indirectly with stress, or just the fact that I was getting older and consequently had a less efficient immune system.

Contemplations on fighting the cancer battle

Cancer, like life itself, is one big, fat crapshoot, a risky venture with no guaranteed outcome. Can the use of metaphor improve the situation and make us feel better? It's a toss-up.

> I see it [the cancer] as something in my body that I'm getting rid of. I don't talk about a battle or a war because I think that sets up that kind of feeling in your body that you're battling something strange inside you.
>
> – Olivia Newton-John

Although using word pictures or imaginative comparisons can give meaning to serious illness, some metaphors lack poetic sensibility. Others are nothing but platitudes. And although it is useful in some cases, e.g. wars, I am tired of the word battle and the winner/loser concept in relation to this disease. (My friend Tim reminded me I felt this way from the early days of hospitalisation). Contemplate the militaristic language regularly used in the media and elsewhere. The patient lost the battle or lost their fight against their cancer, the powerful, highly weaponised and unfeeling enemy within. They failed to win the cancer war. They let the team down; they gave up. They were vanquished (and also vanquished their own cancer cells at the same time).

The whole world seems to be in a state of battle. A quick Google search gives us many examples: the battle against cancer; the corona virus; poverty; dodgy ticket sellers; strong winds; malaria; type 2 diabetes; plastic; over tourism; the devil and second last but not least climate change. My absolute favourite is 'Life is a battle against yourself'. Who the hell is winning that battle?

I admit to being happy to receive words of encouragement from friends and family such as, keep on fighting, don't give up the battle and I am concentrating on positive thoughts every time I think of you. It does help; very much so. It was a fight and a battle of sorts. And in ICU my body certainly engaged in a huge take-over bid with the E. coli bug. However, let's be a bit more adventurous with our terminology when writing books, articles or creating news items in print and on social media. Please give us cancer people a break. How about engaged, duelled, contended or grappled or dealt with cancer? Instead of using fight why not say a challenge, dogfight, provocation, struggle or scrap? I found myself involved in a dogfight with AML. That sounds good – close combat.

I think about Fred's heart disease. Although it was a huge struggle for him no-one called his issues a battle. Is there a battle going on against smallpox, measles or depression? Maybe. Covid 19? Certainly. But have you ever heard of a patient winning the fight against arthritis or eczema? Can a person's body be invaded by hepatitis? Is chemo a form of chemical warfare? If we knew exactly how cancers came about, and if cancers were easily cured, would the terminology change?

Cancer is a disease to be faced, undergone, navigated, put up with or encountered. There is nothing to be ashamed of if the treatment did not work. Somehow the mutated or translocated cells took over your body but they are still part of your body; like the 1950s sci-fi movie *Invasion of the Body Snatchers* in miniature minus the replacement pods lying neatly about the place. Fred has another take on this issue:

> Life threatening illness *is* a battle. When there is a disease in the body there is a battle between bad cells such as bacteria, viruses or cancer cells and healthy cells. Extrapolating from that, the illness becomes a human emotional response. You are in the battle of your life; a battle that must be won. The only options are to fight or succumb. The fighters in your body may fail to win but believing that the illness can be beaten is vital.

I can relate to it myself in the case of GVHD. The donor's lifesaving immune cells *were* in a battle for supremacy over my older and less powerful cells; they were strong and relentless fighters. I have read they were 'mistakenly' doing this but I think they meant it. They were troublemakers, that's for sure. Sometimes they won the melee, sometimes, with the help of drugs, I won. Finally the cells stopped sparring and I guess a truce was declared.

The word journey is also worth a second look. A journey is a trip, a ride, travelling from one place to another. The traveller generally knows their destination and the route they will take. With cancer you have uncertainty and no promise of the outcome. And if cancer is a journey (and, along with my friends, I do use this useful word myself), it is an unpleasant one, full of flat tyres, water in the petrol tank, muggings by strangers and forced diversions to towns offering bad coffee. It is not a journey I want to take again. Let's just say cancer is bigger than a journey. Cancer can be an exploration of sorts, a voyage to inner worlds, and a whole new realm of experience. It is not *necessarily* an opportunity, a character building exercise, a message to make big changes or a chance to appreciate life more. It is not the best thing that has ever happened to me. It is the reverse. Under sufferance I have made the best of it. I have allowed the cancer to define and identify me. For a time my life was all about the disease.

Cancer *does* transform your life, without a doubt. For better, for worse. For richer, for poorer. It can be all consuming. It is an experience that forcibly turns your life right around and forces you to reinvent yourself. No going back, that's for sure.

If life gives you lemons, ask for something else

Self-help books and cancer seem to go hand in glove. Some people are grateful for their cancers because they are given a second chance at life. Others look at it as a chance for personal enlightenment, as a spiritual practice. Some books suggest using positive affirmations such as, I deserve to be happy, I deserve to be loved or I deserve everything the universe has to offer. Call me a cynic but my first thought is, is that so? We all find our own way of coping, but I do find it difficult to relate these affirmations to my own experiences.

A well-intentioned saying – Never give up, never give in – is also meant to inspire those with cancer. Some might disagree but why not give in, take a bromide and collapse in a heap occasionally, or even regularly? Sometimes I don't want to soldier on. Sometimes I do.

In *The Reality Slap*, Russ Harris wrote about one of his

patients whose cancer support group encouraged her to see her illness as a gift. She did not feel this way. Who first conjured up that gift idea? Probably someone spaced out on a cocktail of medicines or a motivational guru who has never had cancer themselves. Cancer is a gift that can keep on giving; it needs to be returned to the sender unopened.

Being reminded that there is always someone worse off than you when you are horribly ill is supposedly a helpful sentence meant to put things in perspective. It is not productive because it downgrades the importance of what the worse off cancer patient is experiencing. There is always someone worse off (or better off) than you – in fact millions and millions of somebodies in many different ways. This includes patients going through AML. How bad do circumstances have to get before you are the worst off person in the waiting room full of people experiencing GVHD symptoms after a transplant?

Welcome to the new normal

One of my mother's favourite sayings whenever my brother Peter and I were mucking around was act normally. I never asked why being normal was better than wrestling Peter to the ground and sitting on him for a while. Since my cancer journey all I have desired is to live a normal life but that state is elusive; it has been incredibly hard to achieve, both for me and the medical team. Cancer is not business as usual. AML has made me feel the opposite of normal. Abnormal white cells, abnormal life.

I came as near to death as you can go in ICU yet didn't have the opportunity to properly test my approach to dying or practice my farewells. One minute I was planning to go home and the next I was unconscious and on life support. Hanging out in ICU is not my idea of an average day at the office and neither is being kept alive artificially with high-tech machinery,

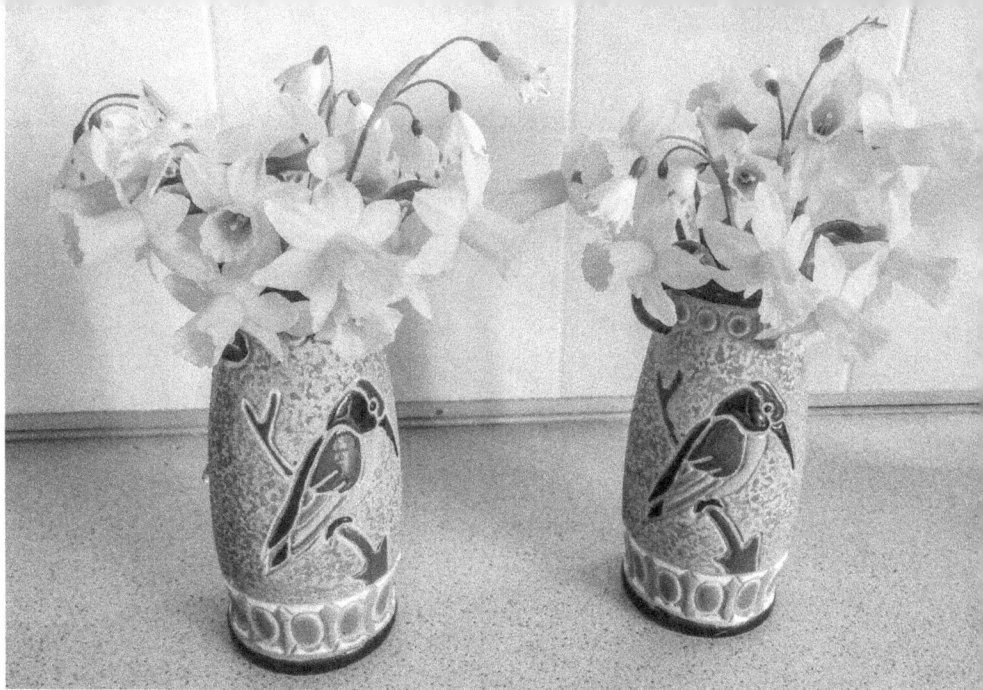

Flowers from my garden in my Amphora vases.

a feeding tube and bucket loads of powerful drugs.

But what is my concept of normal? Physically, normal is waking up and feeling reasonably energetic. Normal is being ready to face the day. Normal is not feeling tired, like a fog or mist is hanging over my brain. Normal is living life without facing big psychic shocks. Normal is the luxury of taking my good health for granted and expecting it will continue. Normal gives an illusion of permanence. Normal is ordinary, and maybe a little boring. Normal is being like other people.

Normal is the past. Being in hospital is not normal. Coughing up blood that looks like coffee grounds and having drug-induced diabetes when you were not previously diabetic is not normal. I can't make any argument for chemo either. Having all my blood levels (and immunity) wiped out and then waiting while they built up again, having my hair fall out, dealing with vomiting and total lack of appetite is not the usual experience. For me, being unable to walk six steps to the door of my room was not normal. Neither was being jealous of every person who could walk about the place without giving it a second thought.

When I came out of the drug-induced coma the dreams/ fantasies came flooding in. Being on a train and cargo ship, made captive by the art dealer, needing to escape from the deadly blood machine, wanting to get to the other side of the fancy glass wall, all had a common theme – overcoming an impenetrable obstacle. I attempted with all my might to reach the normal safe place.

It is not normal to have another person's DNA inside me but over time that DNA has become very much accepted and even loved. I now take it for granted.

So, how to deal with the new world of abnormal? There are no easy answers. I do believe abnormal can become normalised for a short time while ill; a place of equilibrium can be found quite quickly within all the drama and contradictions.

Acceptance and patience are key, but these concepts can't easily be conjured up. Serious mind-work is required, as is taking hope from incremental day-today improvements. I had regular private conversations with myself; some strong words were thrown around. I mixed it up with a bit of coaching and plenty of encouragement.

Come on Cathy, you can get through this. Just hold your breath and put up with the procedure. It is scary but will be over in a minute. You will feel good afterwards.

Stop it! There is no point in wanting to escape from hospital. You know you are in here for weeks. You have to wait for the bloods to build up to normal levels. Each day you can see improvement and everyone cheers for you, so think about that. Be open to change. Stop being a wimp. You don't know if you will die or if the transplant will work. It is going to take time. A great deal of time. Try to get through the day. Check out what the interns are wearing. Look forward to having a shower. Fred will be here soon.

Just accept this could go either way. Resistance is futile. You know you can't control the outcome. You could be well and truly stuffed. But then again a cure might be coming your way

– try and amuse yourself in the meantime.

I never denied the reality of my situation, which turned out to be a positive. And this might sound crazy but, despite being terribly ill, I did not see myself as intrinsically unhealthy. I was just dealing with some powerful leukaemia cells. The rest of my body was okay.

Nowadays a regular life means feeling well, maintaining mental equilibrium, having correct blood readings and not worrying too much about the leukaemia coming back. But to tell you the truth, I'm seriously questioning the concept of normal. Nothing is the way it ought to be and I'm content with that. There is too much change going on in my life to think otherwise.

SOME PRACTICAL ADVICE FOR PATIENTS AND CARERS

Diagnosis

· Listen to your body. If you feel really ill and the sick feeling does not dissipate, don't hesitate to seek medical attention. You know your own body well so let it guide you

· Take the medical advice via Dr Google with a large grain of salt, especially when googling symptoms and survival statistics. Headings such as: What causes AML? – 6 Shocking Facts and Is leukaemia a death sentence? can give you an unnecessary scare. Check out Anonymous Nurse: Please Stop Using 'Dr. Google' to Diagnose Your Symptoms at https://www.healthline.com/health/please-stop-using-doctor-google-dangerous

· The initial diagnosis of your illness may not be the correct one. Doctors are not infallible and may not be familiar with rare diseases. If in doubt obtain a second or even a third opinion.

Fear of needles and hospital procedures

· Fear of hypodermic needles or injections affects over 20% of the population to some extent. It can be life-threatening when the sufferer avoids seeking much needed medical attention. Remember, procedures involving needles generally do not hurt much, if at all. The fear of the procedure is out of proportion to the reality

· Support is at hand. Try hypnotherapy, relaxation techniques and Cognitive-Behavioural Therapy (CBT).

Cancer education

· If you are diagnosed with blood cancer it is worth getting educated for what lies ahead; to get a grip on what is happening inside your body and what the treatment options are. It can be quite frightening to know these facts but to use a cliché, knowledge is power. Be as well-informed as possible, take an active role in your care and advocate for your own life

· Information on blood and other cancers is abundant; make sure the source you access is a well-known and respected authority such as the Leukaemia Foundation, the Cancer Council or Mayo Clinic

· In hospital you can discuss any issues with the medical staff. You will also receive brochures outlining each stage of the process as you approach that milestone.

Dealing with ICU

Visiting a patient in ICU can be very confronting. Patients can become agitated and confused due to the illness or the medication given. They may hallucinate and become convinced others are deceiving them. This should improve as the patient recovers. If the patient has been given sedatives, it can take hours or even days for the weaning process to kick in. The patient may be drowsy and confused as they come out of sedation. I know I was. Practical information can be found on the Intensive Care Foundation website: https://www.intensivecarefoundation.org.au/visiting-a-patient-in-the-icu/

Communications and spreading the word about your illness

· Decide who you want to tell about your illness, if anyone. Remember, keeping it secret can be difficult and exhausting. It can be even worse if some people know and others do not. A great deal of love and support will come your way once your family, friends and colleagues hear of your plight

· Work out a way of communicating with everyone that works for you all. Group texts or emails from you or your carer are a sensible, time saving way of keeping everyone in the loop. Repeating the same information over and over will be draining. As a patient undergoing chemo you can feel debilitated – constant exhaustion and regular severe nausea being high on the list. Families get frightened too and then they look to the patient for reassurance and love. It might be necessary to halt visits for periods of time in order to provide a peaceful time to just lie in bed and not talk at all.

Practical tips for coping in hospital

· Jazz up your room and bed but remember – no flowers or real plants, only fake

· Say goodbye to a good night's sleep or the chance to dream. You will be lucky to get an uninterrupted four-hour shut eye at any one time. Nap time between procedures, meals, observations and all the other hospital business will become precious time

· Don't yearn too much for the outside world. Try to accept that the hospital will be your home for some time yet

· Grab a pair of headphones and listen to your favourite music tracks or watch a show on your laptop

- It is challenging but get used to being attached to tubes and equipment 24/7 for a few days and maybe longer, depending on chemo delivery, hydration requirements etc.

- Accept that you will feel frightened, angry, helpless, forlorn or envious. It is important to acknowledge all your feelings, negative and positive. You don't have to put on a brave face to protect your loved ones from worry – unless you want to. Don't be afraid to ask for help. And say so if you feel overloaded with helpful advice from family and friends

- Visitors – you don't need to bombard your charge or friend with idle chit chat, questions or information. Just simply being present, providing quietness and peace, can be very reassuring. Just hang out, you don't need to change the way you act and speak, try to treat them as you normally would. Don't worry about what to say or write when a loved one has cancer. Clichés or platitudes are hard to avoid.

Gifts for the patient

All gifts are welcome and of course your choice will depend on the patient. Reading materials were welcome to me but it was hard to concentrate on a large book; magazines were mentally easier to digest. Consider a hospital TV or internet subscription. Colouring books? A pashmina or small soft blanket? Green tea? I welcomed hats and beanies for warmth after hair loss, woollen socks, quality soap, hand cream without too strong a fragrance, lip balm, a sheepskin rug and fruit baskets. Keeping up with everyone via their social media posts, emails, cards and photographs also helped to keep my spirits up.

Tablet taking

· At home it is easy to lose track of what tablets you have taken, or if you have forgotten to take them altogether. Use a tablet holder with compartments for each day of the week and sections for morning, afternoon and night

· If you find large tablets hard to swallow, ask if a smaller version is available

· Reading the detailed information sheets found inside the box of drugs can be worrying, especially the often huge list of side effects. Remember, most probably won't affect you and are listed in part to cover the potential liabilities of drug companies

· Be informed about what drugs you are taking; your prescriptions, amounts, side effects and cost. Some chemists are more expensive than others. Go generic if available. If you are a public patient, check that your prescription does not say private patient as it will cost you more. And don't forget to check the number of repeats remaining and the validity date, especially if you are planning a trip overseas or interstate

· The traveller's exemption allows people entering (and leaving) Australia to carry their medicines and medical devices with them (in accompanied baggage) for their own personal use or the use by an immediate family member who is travelling with them, up to a limit of three months' supply. Carry sufficient prescription medications to cover your time overseas and leave the medicines in their original packaging with dispensing label intact. Don't forget to obtain a letter from your doctor listing the name and dosage of medications you are taking for your condition. You do not need special permission to bring insulin with you for personal use

· Unused drugs can be taken to your pharmacist for disposal.

Allogenic transplant

If you are offered an allogenic (donor) transplant, read up, seek advice from your specialist and consider the risks carefully. Stem cell transplants are a complex business. They are expensive and require a great deal of preparation and time from yourself and hospital staff, both before and after the procedure. It may not work and there is a good chance you will need to deal with symptoms of GVHD, either acute, chronic or both.

Managing Appetite Loss

My mouth become quite sensitive after chemo; the nurses gave me ice chips to suck on along with a mouthwash to use. My appetite was low. I lost interest in many of my favourite foods and craved bland foods such as custard. However my sense of taste returned to normal over time. The dietitians pointed out that good nutrition was a significant aid to recovery. It was essential to stay well hydrated and I needed to eat more to keep up my energy levels, lower the risk of infection and heal faster.

Exercise

After spending a long period of time in bed, it takes a while to regain balance, strength and mobility. Exercise as much as you can both in and out of hospital. You can do it. Use light weights for strength training, even in your hospital bed. Ride a stationary bicycle or take a daily walk. Do yoga.

The Cancer Council Victoria website has some good tips on exercise: https://www.cancervic.org.au/living-with-cancer/exercise/exercise-overview

Therapy

Seek professional assistance if depression or severe anxiety persists, happens without any particular reason or makes it hard to cope. Medicare can help with the cost of a registered mental health professional. Check out the Human Services website: https://www.humanservices.gov.au/individuals/subjects/whats-covered-medicare/mental-health-care-and-medicare

Colonoscopies

The National Bowel Cancer Screening Program is a population based screening program that aims to help detect bowel cancer early and reduce the number of Australians who die each year from the disease. Eligible people, starting at age 50 and continuing to age 74 (without symptoms) are invited by mail to complete a simple test kit at home and send it to the program's pathology laboratory for analysis. There is no cost involved. The test involves taking a tiny sample of faeces which is tested in a pathology laboratory. The test can detect tiny amounts of blood in faeces which may be a sign of cancer or polyps. Just do it! http://www.cancerscreening.gov.au/internet/screening/publishing.nsf/Content/bowel-screening-1

Coping with life after remission

· One of the major challenges during treatment and recovery is that life around you continues on regardless. And this can be confronting when you feel permanently tired, sick and emotionally fragile. Friends and family might become sick, or even may die, as was my experience. This can be hugely difficult to manage, and you may need professional assistance to get through all of this. But also, all the little things, like paying bills, shopping, housekeeping, cooking and eating need to be dealt with. Tensions can build up and small things can take on extra significance, let alone the big things. Don't worry that you will appear weak and are not coping. You will be struggling from time to time. Ask for help. It is OK and people will understand

- Recovery from cancer will lead to unexpected lifestyle changes. Be open to change and see where it leads

- Connect with a relevant, supportive Facebook group where you can network with other people impacted by cancer

- If you have some ready cash, feel up to it, and your doctor approves, take the opportunity to travel. Go overseas or interstate, visit friends and family. Visit a nearby town for lunch or go to the beach. Try to take a holiday from your illness.

Type 2 Diabetes

- Check out the ABC's Catalyst program in which Nutritionist Dr Joanna McMillan is on a mission to help stem the onslaught of type 2 diabetes, devising a personalised program to help four Australians on the brink of developing the chronic illness. http://www.abc.net.au/catalyst/stories/4888637.htm

- If you have (or develop) diabetes or another condition which may affect your driving ability, you are required to notify the relevant transport authority in your state

- People registered with the National Diabetes Services Scheme are able to access services, support and subsidised diabetes products to assist them to self-manage their life with diabetes. https://www.ndss.com.au/services/

Fear of the cancer returning

- The fear of the cancer returning can be overwhelming. This is totally understandable. Accept your feelings but try not to worry too much or speculate on what may or may not happen in the future. For helpful advice read the Cancer Council's web page *Fear of the Cancer Coming Back*. https://www.cancercouncil.com.au/15291/b1000/living-well-after-cancer-45/living-well-after-cancer-fear-of-recurrence/

- Don't be afraid to talk with your family about the kind of funeral you would like. It is better than having to second guess all the ceremony details if and when you have departed.

The natural approach

- For the cancer patient everything about a hospital environment is artificial, from the lighting to the air you are breathing. If you are at all mobile, or can access a wheel chair, spend time outdoors. Stimulate all your senses. Rebuild your vitamin D levels. Nature has extraordinary healing powers. Along with music, it is the best medicine

- The soft hospital bandages wrapped around the elbow after a blood test make excellent plant ties for tomatoes and other veggies

- Use organic products and techniques in your garden or on the farm. If a product is labelled Poison definitely consider using a less toxic alternative

- Plant drifts of indigenous and native plants to attract birds, bees and insects

- Grow your own herbs, fruit and vegetables. Even a few pots on a balcony can provide you with some delicious tomatoes, parsley, lettuce etc.

- Support local producers. Buy fresh foods at farmers markets. Buy organic foods where budget permits

- Carry water in a recyclable bottle, not plastic. Drink filtered water or water from your tap.

Learn about other experiences of blood cancer

- Have your thoughts provoked. You are not alone. While writing *Life Blood* I deliberately avoided reading any books specifically about the little c. I wanted to ensure my ideas came from inside me, not second-hand or under the influence of other people's ideas. It was exciting to then delve into other narratives, including Evan Handler's unrelenting *Time on Fire: My Comedy of Terrors*, golfer Jarrod Lyle's *My Story*, and Kirsty Everett's moving childhood experience *Honey Blood*. Paul Kalanithi's memoir *When Breath Becomes Air* is a profound insight into how a neurosurgeon diagnosed with inoperable lung cancer dealt with life as a patient and new father. He faced his own death without self-pity. Siddhatha Mukherjee was awarded the Pulitzer Prize for *The Emperor of all Maladies: a biography of cancer*, quoted by the *Independent* as 'A tale of hopes, dreams and pincer-sharp disappointment.'

- For useful advice for patients and their supporters check out the free e-book *Caring for Someone with Cancer* at https://www.cancer.org.au. Read Jo Spicer's book *Survive and Thrive! How Cancer Saves Lives* or *Talking about cancer: laying bare the emotions* by Lib Heyward at https://www.urevolution.com/talking-about-cancer-laying-bare-emotions/.

Financials

- For peace of mind take out Ambulance Victoria membership. Emergency medical transport is costly, especially if an air ambulance is required as this cost is not covered by Medicare

- A helpful tip regarding referrals from general practitioners to specialists. If you need ongoing treatment for a health condition, your GP can write up an indefinite referral, saving you time, effort and expense. You do not need to organise a referral every year

- Manage multiple medical appointments by printing notifications and referrals and keeping them in a folder. Immediately write doctors' appointments into a calendar which is prominently placed on your wall for easy reference

- Make sure you are informed of the cost, if any, before X-rays, CT scans etc. are taken, not afterwards

- Ensure your will is up to date and consider creating a medical and/or legal power of attorney

- Organisations such as Ronald McDonald House can assist families of seriously ill children and the Leukaemia Foundation provides low cost or free accommodation and transport to blood cancer patients and their carers

- Sign up for a fundraiser such as Dry July or World's Greatest Shave Volunteer your time and expertise

- Family and friends – offer practical day to day support. Drive your loved one to outpatient and medical appointments. Take care of their children, deliver some delicious home cooked meals to their home or bedside if allowed or offer to do some housework or gardening. Start a Go Fund Me page if their finances are tight.

Register as a donor

If you reside in Australia, are between 18 and 45 years old, in good health, meet the eligibility criteria and are prepared to donate for anyone in the world, there is every possibility you may save the life of someone with blood cancer. Call the Australian Red Cross on 13 14 95 to make an appointment to donate blood and join the Australian Bone Marrow Donor Registry. https://www.abmdr.org.au/

USEFUL CONTACTS

The Alfred Hospital, Caulfield Hospital
and Sandringham Hospital
https://www.alfredhealth.org.au/

Leukaemia Foundation
https://www.leukaemia.org.au/

Intensive Care Foundation
https://www.intensivecarefoundation.org.au/

PPDB Pesticide Properties Database.
University of Hertfordshire
https://sitem.herts.ac.uk/aeru/ppdb/en/index.htm

Rare Cancers Australia
http://www.rarecancers.org.au/

Diabetes Institute
https://www.diabetesaustralia.com.au/

National Diabetes Services Scheme
https://www.ndss.com.au/services/

Geoff Beats Leukemia
https://geoffbeatsleukemia.com/

Peter MacCallum Cancer Centre
https://www.petermac.org/

Olivia Newton-John Cancer Wellness and Research Centre
https://www.onjcancercentre.org/

Australian Bone Marrow Donor Registry
https://www.abmdr.org.au/

Confronting stories from an ICU nurse
https://thefootnotes.com.au/nursing-uncut/

Challenge: Supporting Kids with Cancer
https://www.challenge.org.au/

Mayo Clinic
https://www.mayoclinic.org/

Cancer Council Australia
https://www.cancer.org.au/

Skin Health Institute
https://www.skinhealthinstitute.org.au/

Australian Red Cross Lifeblood
https://www.lifeblood.com.au/

Better Health Channel
https://www.betterhealth.vic.gov.au/

CanTeen
https://www.canteen.org.au/

Beyond Blue
https://www.beyondblue.org.au/

FURTHER READING

Arikawa, Hiro, *The Travelling Cat Chronicle*, Transworld Publishers, London, 2017

Benjamin, Briony, *Life is Tough But So Are You: How to rise to the challenge when things go pear-shaped*, Murdoch Books Pty Ltd, 2021

Ehrenreich, Barbara, *Smile or Die: How Positive Thinking Fooled America & The World*, Granta Publications, London 2009

Everett, Kirsty, *Honey Blood: A memoir*, Harper Collins Publishers, Sydney NSW, 2021

Goodhart, Frances and Atkins, Lucy, T*he Cancer Survivor's Companion: practical ways to cope with your feelings after cancer*, Piatkus, London, 2011.

Handler, Evan, *Time on Fire: My Comedy of Terrors*. Souvenir Press, London, 1996.

Harris, Russell, *The Happiness Trap: stop struggling, start living*, Exisle Publishing Ltd, Wollombi, N.S.W, 2007

Harris, Russell, *The Reality Slap: How to find fulfilment when life hurts*, Exisle Publishing Ltd, Wollombi, N.S.W, 2011

Steve Harris, *The Prince and The Assassin: Australia's First Royal Tour and Portent of World Terror*, Melbourne Books, Melbourne 2017

Hyde, A.D., *The Leukaemia Diaries: Seeing the Funnier Side of Cancer*, Balboa Press, Bloomington, Indiana, 2020

Kalanithi, Paul, *When Breath Becomes Air*, Random House, New York, 2016

Komen, Josh, *The Wind at My Back: A memoir of cancer, love and endurance*, Mary Egan Publishing, New Zealand, 2019

Lyle, Jarrod with Hayes, Mark and Blake, Martin, *My Story*, Lake Press, Hawthorn, Victoria 2019

Mukherjee, Siddhartha, *The Emperor of all Maladies: a biography of cancer*, Scribner, New York, 2010

Ryan, Luke, *A Funny Thing Happened on the Way to Chemo: a memoir of getting cancer -twice!* Affirm Press, South Melbourne, Victoria, 2014

Sales, Leigh, *Any Ordinary Day*, Hamish Hamilton Australia, Camberwell, Victoria, 2018

Spicer, Jo, *Survive and Thrive! How Cancer Saves Lives: Inspiring Stories of Courageous Cancer Thrivers*, Crown Kent, Sydney, NSW, 2019

Sontag, Susan, *Illness as Metaphor*, Farrar, Strauss and Giroux, New York, c1978

Watt, Ben, Patient: *The True Story of a Rare Illness*, Bloomsbury Publishing Plc, London, 2014

ACKNOWLEDGMENTS

There are so many people to thank. It takes a village to save and maintain a life.

First I want to express my deep gratitude to The Alfred Hospital's medical team directly involved in my long-term care – Professor David Curtis, nursing specialists Georgia, Danielle, Bianca and Dr Trish Wright. Thank you so much for your ongoing support. Although I am one patient of many, The Alfred is my second home and you always make me feel deserving of your attention.

Thanks also to the many medical professionals and staff members whose paths have crossed mine both at The Alfred and elsewhere, from the GPs, nurses and specialists to the receptionists, cleaners, phlebotomists and pharmacists, with a special thank you to Susan Mason at the Alfred Foundation.

Recognition and appreciation don't seem like strong enough words to use when it comes to acknowledging my family and close friends. You have all been my knights in shining armour.

Thank you for continuing to ask how the writing is proceeding, for reading the manuscript and advising on book content and the cover, for allowing me to quote you, for the testimonials.

For all the gifts, best wishes and emails, for the visits, the warm beds and the many meals enjoyed, for the encouraging and amusing Facebook posts, for the laughs.

For giving advice and allowing me to offer the same, for understanding when I didn't feel well, for being a part of my life.

My families: Peter, John, Danielle, Ben, Christopher, Stephanie, Maria, Robert and Glenys, Adrian and Marianne, Tini, Winny and Jan, Denise and family.

The extended family: Tim, Ronda and Sharna, Duré, Damian.

The Xavier connection: Ana, Con, Sonya, Bob, Sam and Jane.

The gardening connection: Janine, Bronwyn, Fran and Richard.

Great friends: Jim and Paulette, Mansook, James and Rebecca, Tom and Jenny, Frank, Julian and Simone, Sandi, Alexandra, Trisha and Gary, Annemaree, Viviana, Karen and Frank.

Fellow AML survivor Geoff and wife Jan.

To Dr Russ Harris for writing the Foreword for the book and for his and Natasha's ongoing advice and friendship.

To my wonderful editor Amanda McMahon for your insights, your expertise and for keeping me on track.

To Julie Postance from iinspire media, my knowledgeable and generous independent publishing mentor.

To Sophie, of Sophie White Design, thank you for making my book look so good.

And finally to my best friend and life partner Fred, my heartfelt thanks for your endless patience, care and support. There are many years still to enjoy.

ABOUT THE AUTHOR

Cathy Koning likes to re-invent herself. She briefly worked as a secondary school teacher after graduating with an arts degree from La Trobe University. As a theatre photographer she captured over thirty productions at the Last Laugh Theatre Restaurant in Melbourne from the late 1970's and toured Europe with Nigel Triffitt's *Momma's Little Horror Show* as costume coordinator and photographer. After a stint as a cinema publicist she founded a successful gardening business and then ran a Sustainable Communities Program for two rural shires.

Everything changed in 2012 with a leukaemia diagnosis. During her long recovery Cathy turned her hand to writing and *Dainty Diva*, the biography of Dorothy Rudder, a Sydney soprano and vaudeville artist, was the outcome. *Life Blood*, the story of her cancer journey, gave her the chance to reflect on what it meant to be confronted by a frightening diagnosis and the comfort she found in family, friends and access to an excellent public health system. She is currently researching her next book about a notorious American con-man.

Dainty Diva can be downloaded free of charge from my website cathykoningwriter.com. Theatre historian and author Frank van Straten kindly provided the following endorsement.

What an exciting pleasure to meet the delightful Dorothy Rudder! With warmth and expertise Cathy Koning evokes Dorothy's long stage, concert and radio career and the theatre greats with whom she worked. With its treasure trove of fascinating illustrations, Dainty Diva is an invaluable exploration of a now largely forgotten world of Australian and international show business. I heartily recommend it.

www.ingramcontent.com/pod-product-compliance
Lightning Source LLC
Chambersburg PA
CBHW030242030426
42336CB00009B/218